ELECTIVE MUTISM

NEUROPSYCHOLOGY AND COGNITION

VOLUME 5

The purpose of the Neuropsychology and Cognition series is to bring out volumes that promote understanding in topics relating brain and behavior. It is intended for use by both clinicians and research scientists in the fields of neuropsychology, cognitive psychology, psycholinguistics, speech and hearing, as well as education. Examples of topics to be covered in the series would relate to memory, language acquisition and breakdown, reading, attention, developing and aging brain. By addressing the theoretical, empirical, and applied aspects of brain-behavior relationships, this series will try to present the information in the fields of neuropsychology and cognition in a coherent manner.

The titles published in this series are listed at the end of this volume.

NORMAN H. HADLEY

Department of Educational Psychology, Memorial University of Newfoundland,
St. John's, Newfoundland, Canada

Elective Mutism:
A Handbook for Educators,
Counsellors and
Health Care Professionals

KLUWER ACADEMIC PUBLISHERS
DORDRECHT / BOSTON / LONDON

Library of Congress Cataloging-in-Publication Data

Hadley, N. H. (Norman Harvey)
    Elective mutism   a handbook for educators, counsellors, and
  health care professionals / by Norman H. Hadley.
        p.   cm. -- (Neuropsychology and cognition . 5)
    Includes bibliographical references and indexes.
    ISBN 0-7923-2418-8 (hb   alk. paper)
    1. Mutism, Elective.   I. Title.   II. Series.
    [DNLM   1. Mutism--in infancy & childhood.   2. Mutism--psychology.
  3. Mutism--therapy.   4. Psychotherapy--methods.   5. Social
  Environment.   W1 NE342DG v. 5 / WM 475 H 1312e 1994]
  RJ506.M87H3   1994
  618.92'84--dc20
  DNLM/DLC
  for Library of Congress   93-27859

ISBN 0-7923-2418-8

Published by Kluwer Academic Publishers,
P.O. Box 17, 3300 AA Dordrecht, The Netherlands.

Kluwer Academic Publishers incorporates the publishing programmes
of D. Reidel, Martinus Nijhoff, Dr W. Junk and MTP Press.

Sold and distributed in the U.S.A. and Canada
by Kluwer Academic Publishers,
101 Philip Drive, Norwell, MA 02061, U.S.A.

In all other countries, sold and distributed
by Kluwer Academic Publishers Group,
P.O. Box 322, 3300 AH Dordrecht, The Netherlands.

Printed on acid-free paper

Printed in the Netherlands

Lovingly Dedicated to My Wife, Catherine

TABLE OF CONTENTS

FOREWORD

Undeniably, language is at the core of human existence. Merleau-Ponty (1945) posited that thought and language are one – cognition being language; language, cognition. Although such a categorical stance can be challenged from a number of theoretical perspectives as dogmatic and nonveridical, the critical role of language in humanness is irrefutable. It is what defines and distinguishes creatures at the apex of the phylogenetic scale. The fact that cognition predates verbal fluency and can take various nonverbal forms does not diminish the pivotal role of language – it is a functional requisite, an imperative. More than a mere vehicle to express thought, it transforms, modifies and shapes much of cognition. It cannot be trivialized.

On many grounds man is capably rivalled by lower forms of existence – the gazelle is more graceful; the lion is stronger; the cheetah is fleeter. It is through his use of symbols that man usurps the ascendant position. Cassirer in *Essay on Man* (1946) described man as *animal symbolicum*, the animal that creates symbols and a symbolic world. Through language, humans transcend time and are able to describe events temporally removed – to reflect on the past, to conjecture the future. With words man can paint pictures, muse and dream, embrace and console, persuade and corrupt, educate and be educated. Language is a preferred performatory domain, nowhere more than in Western Civilization.

The direction of ontological development is toward a more extensive and elaborate use of symbols. With maturity comes the ability to deal with abstraction, to function independent of the physically present, to introspect, to achieve meta-awareness, to generate strategies and solutions. Language is *not just another* of many attributes which help to define the course of human development.

Humans vary in their facility with language. They are not equally fluent nor equally capable of exploiting the power of language. Some are demagogues and some are poets; others struggle inarticulately with language attempts. But most strive to use language. It is as if language must emerge, as if it "must out." Even the most developmentally delayed individuals try to find expression through language, albeit simplistic and arduously generated in many cases. Those who are denied language or are restricted in its use are described as disabled, delayed or handicapped. In such cases education becomes a catalyst for language production, an inexhaustible search for what will work, a mustering of resources to obviate dependency and social ostracism. Compensatory and augmentative communication systems are viewed as a last resort. Yet, some *choose to be silent.*

Norman Hadley probes the complexity of silence use in his challenging work. If it were a simple task anyone could have completed it. Entering a maelstrom of theoretical ambiguity and conflict, he critically examines the amorphous elective mutism phenomenon. The behavior pattern of those who elect to be "silence users" portrays disruption in a primary (if not the most critical) development task – achieving access to an increasingly complex world of symbols. To search out, integrate and make meaningful strides toward a holistic framework from diverse literature comprised of n = 1 case studies and small sample research is both an onerous and formidable task. The area defies broad brush strokes.

In the initial segment of the manuscript Professor Hadley focuses upon the complexity of silence. He provides a unique dissertation on silence as an aspect of communication, capable of either a positive or negative valence. It is intriguing to consider silence as an occurrence with many possible meanings rather than as a lull or "dead spot" in conversation, an awkward temporal spacing between the words of a speaker who is unfamiliar with a topic, or two speakers who are unfamiliar with each other. The common tendency to cancel silences with "ahs," "ums" and suchlike in Western communication speaks of our discomfort with it and the tendency to view it pejoratively. Silence is *not* our custom.

To ascribe multiple meanings to silence is to validate it as a complex facet of communication – chilling silence, emphatic silence, dogmatic silence, defiant silence, elective silence. Hadley's detailed study of silence is more than an interesting preamble. Rather than being tangential to the main thrust of the book, the discourse presents a logical starting point, a base-line. From within the general context of silence in its many forms, both pathological and productive, the author sharpens the focus to center upon a specific negative use of silence, the central tenent of the elective mutism concept.

As I read through Hadley's writing I found myself struggling (as I sensed he had) with a basic question concerning what is aberrant and what is justifiable and responsible with regard to the use of silence. In essence: Where and how does one define limits for the continuum of "normal" silence usage? How much distance is there between the shy, reticent and untoward child and one who requires etiological definition and intervention? The two most recurrent (although certainly not the only) etiological themes presented in the book are that elective mutism is driven by *fear reduction* in many instances, and that it has a *manipulative attention-seeking* basis in many others. These theoretical orientations deserve comment – as separate entities, as they relate to each other, and as they relate to other etiological possibilities.

Within the context of elective mutism as a fear-reducing mechanism, it strikes me that when an environment is so stressing and hurtful that it prompts a child to retreat into silence, we must be careful as to where we assign the pathology. Perhaps such children are hyper-resilient, capable of protecting and sustaining themselves in the face of dire adversity. In such cases, the environment might be viewed as dysfunctional, rather than the child who is coping with it through silence.

Often in abusive families and classrooms children do not risk verbal involvement. Ray Helfer (1981), with reference to psychological child abuse, described such "muting" or denial of self-expression as "developmental erosion." What must be remembered is that while the individual episode of silence use might be viewed as an effective coping response, the net effect of prolonged use of silence as a defense from fear is devastating and can create more than superficial problems for even the most resilient child. For other children, the fear which drives their mutism is in a true sense psychogenic, a different entity, fostered by a desire to escape from an innocuous or imagined stimulus.

Silence users classified as "attention-seeking manipulative" are presented in the literature as standing in contrast to those whose mutism is fear-inspired. Although the basic manifestation – *silence* – is congruent for the groups, critical differences in behavior often help to distinguish between the groups, making the origin of silence identifiable. However, a definitive etiological classification is not always possible. Briefly consider elective mutism within the theoretical frame of reference of *hostility theory*. Within this orientation, a child's use of silence may be interpreted in terms of at least two simultaneous and compatible elements: (1) prolonged silence as a potent weapon to direct against others (manipulative) and, (2) reduction of the risk of punishment which active aggression might prompt (fear-inspired).

Hadley believes that a parsimonious two-group approach to elective mutism – *fear-based* and *attention-seeking manipulative* – does not realistically reflect its many *in viva* persona. Accordingly, he proposes that such groups be envisioned as pole positions on a causal continuum rather than as the dichotomous entities presented in many research and treatment orientations. In agreement, I would underscore that the concept defies easy explanation and would suggest that a linear model might need to be replaced by a multidimensional matrix capable of accommodating the variety of possible interacting causal factors. It is conceivable that many factors such as symbiotic attachment, sound-of-one's-voice speech phobia, and manipulative behavior might coexist in a challenging conundrum of silence use. The possible interrelationships are infinite. Clearly, some instances of silence are more easily managed theoretically than others; a large segment must always be viewed as n = 1 studies. The conjoint impact of unique clusters of elements (such as trauma, observational learning, and aversive stimuli) will continue to muddy the waters for both understanding and helping.

Historically, research literature in the area has been descriptive, the presentation of specific cases with attendant characteristics. The area has suffered from a paucity of systematic theory building. Hadley has made inroads. At the very least, he has placed all the pieces of the puzzle on the table.

At the outset I described what to me is the dynamic role of language – to empower, to activate, to frame cognition. It is important to note that with elective mutism the child does not deny or reject language totally. It is behavior which is voluntary, "elective" being the key word. The extent to which language is withheld varies from one individual to another as does the context for silence. Frequently it is failure to verbalize within the educational setting that defines the problem. Such learners forgo linguistic engagement, the life-blood of education.

My belief is that education is a dialogue in which individuals help to create each other. Each time I teach a course at university, whether it be in New Brunswick, Alberta or Newfoundland, I am changed through the process – sometimes slightly, sometimes markedly. My students help to create me as hopefully I do them. James Baldwin in *Tell Me How Long the Train's Been Gone* (1968) succinctly defined the reciprocal process of education involving a more mature person and one with less experience. Without specific reference to "formal education," he captured its essence:

If it is true, as I suspect, that people turn to each other in the hope of being created by each other then it is absolutely true that the uncreated young turn, to be created, toward their elders. Thus, whoever has been invested with the power of enchantment is guilty of something more base than treachery whenever he fails to exercise the power on which the yet-to-be-created, as helplessly as newborn birds, depend. (p. 82)

Within this creative process, elective mutism is a debilitating intrusion, a developmental hiatus having varying degrees of severity. Recognizing its potential to render the child dysfunctional, Professor Hadley addresses the treatment aspect of the phenomenon with commitment. *Elective Mutism* is more than a heuristic quest for theoretical closure. Although it is that in one sense, it is also a source for treatment alternatives and directions. Having acknowledged that being electively mute is dysfunctional, it is necessary at some point to confront the problem irrespective of its genesis. Hadley's grounding in special education theory is reflected in his general disposition toward intervention – progression from a less restrictive to a more restrictive technique only to the extent warranted, and only after the less aversive method has been tried. Advice aligning with standard "good practice" is pervasive in chapter components which are geared toward the pragmatics of intervention.

It is clear from Hadley's summation that positive reinforcement approaches have much to offer given their reported intervention effectiveness. But this does not obviate other treatment methods. Dr. Hadley's wide-ranging professional background is inextricably part of his treatment orientation. He does not close the door on unique and innovative strivings. To him, the therapist must not be a carpenter who attempts to repair all damage, including broken windows, while limited to a saw or hammer tool choice.

Hadley presents a strong case for considering the various forms of expressive therapy as treatment options. Particularly convincing are his arguments for their value as a means to establish therapist-client rapport during the initial stage of therapy, and later, as worthwhile conjunctions between no communication and verbal exchange. The entire gamut of creative art forms from finger-painting to drama to dance are suggested as possible precursors to appropriate verbal behavior. Having expertise in the area of "art therapy" lends credence to Dr. Hadley's assessment that much more than token recognition must be afforded expressive therapies in the treatment of electively mute clients.

The data presented in tabular format throughout the book (surveying everything from first communications during therapy to follow-up results) represents an exhaustive examination of primary sources. I doubt that one would discover another compilation of information as extensive as this in the field. Given the amorphous nature of reported research findings, Hadley's effort to superimpose order is laudable.

Along the same line, with a view toward usability, the comprehensive scale developed for use in the interview situation should be a welcome tool. Drawing from varied sources, as well as personal experience, Hadley has forged a much needed instrument which will undoubtedly replace earlier hit-and-miss approaches. Thoroughness is its strength.

Throughout the book there is a sensitive recognition that children *are children*, not a chain of paper doll clients neatly defined under the elective mutism rubric. Pervasive is the author's sustained view that the child *as a person* must not be lost during the treatment process whether it be psychodynamic, behavior management based or whatever. As noted in the book, "elective mutism can have other impacts which are as important as the deterioration of academic performance."

It is this that makes Hadley's work so worthwhile; succinctly, it is his willingness to assign priority to the individual as center of the therapeutic process. It is the backdrop for inter-modal therapy. As homogeneity is not assumed among silence users, a singular restrictive treatment focus is not proposed.

It is interesting to speculate concerning the disproportionate female:male ratio cited in the literature with regard to elective mutism. At first glance this appears quite enigmatic given that the opposite is the case with the preponderance of learning disabilities such as dyslexia (6 boys:1 girl) which relates to language as well. Perhaps the sex differences in elective mutism mirror the male dominance generally indicated in conversations between the sexes – i.e., turn-taking and speech interruption patterns. Subjectively, I feel that silence has been demanded and reinforced historically as a central part of female family and social roles. Perhaps for too long – but this is another issue.

Hadley's writing provokes one to speculate concerning the number of individuals who go through life as unacknowledged silence users. How many choose silence as a defense or recoil into silence for want of a sympathetic listener? I believe that there are many for whom speech is perfunctory, elective, and indifferent. As the author points out, "only silence which is troublesome for others receives attention and correction." Perhaps there is a sister parallel phenomenon to elective mutism which has its roots in the fast-paced rivalry which we have come to view as life. *Elective hearing-loss* merits study.

This book has not been completed with ease or in haste. Norman Hadley can be found in his writing – sensitive, rigorous, and lucid. I am very pleased to have been asked to contribute.

Wayne C. Nesbit, Ph.D.
Chair, Special Education
Memorial University of Newfoundland

PREFACE

If readers are looking for the development of a single argument or thesis, they will not find it in my book. The book approaches the topic of elective mutism with a multidimensional focus. I would like to make a point or two about the style of this book. Some aspects are penned in a scholarly style while other facets are penned in the language of human feelings rather than in behavioristic words and operational definitions. In introducing this book, I would like to explain how I became interested in elective mutism and what sustained me in following this work to completion. The preparation of my book extended over several years and since I am the sole author it was sometimes a lonely and silent task. Christopher Alexander, in the *Timeless Way of Building*, refers to an inner sense of aliveness that best describes my experience while writing this book. My book is more than a compendium of findings. I have identified and critiqued a number of major issues. In addition, I have included my personal reflections on the process, and have attempted to delineate specific problems for research.

There are many reasons why I wrote the book. The first relates to my curiosity about elective mutism as a pathological response. Indeed, this curiosity soon widened to include other aspects of silence which play a role in human communication. Almost without exception, the reference list in published studies of elective mutism does not include a single citation about the use of silence in everyday communication or the significance of silence in nonverbal communication. To study elective mutism without considering the important context of the use and significance of silence in communication leads to a narrow focus on the behavior problem. The more I studied the factors of silence in human behavior, the more I was motivated to include and expand on this backdrop for elective mutism. The problem of elective mutism only becomes meaningful if it is studied within the context of the day-to-day use of silence. There are many "sounds of silence" which are a part of day-to-day communication. Elective mutism is only one silence-related communication problem. There are people who talk too much and there are people who are accused of talking too much. Silence based on gender differences is especially important because elective mutism is one of the few behavior problems of childhood in which the incidence is greater among females than males.

The encouraging feedback which I received from the participants who attended my presentation on Elective Mutism in Children and Adolescents

at the 1987 conference of the Canadian Association of Speech-Language
Pathologists and Audiologists also empowered me to write the book. Since
I am an enthusiastic learner, I am eager to hear from clinicians who are
working with electively mute children and from previously electively mute
individuals.

ASSESSMENT OF ELECTIVELY MUTE BEHAVIOR

An assessment instrument for elective mutism is included in Chapter 13.
Questions may be selected which coincide with the specific characteristics of the silence user role. I anticipate, therefore, that the clinician will
benefit from a convenient source of questions which might be used in
pretreatment assessment and in monitoring intervention effects. Data
obtained on specific questions – for example before the intervention, at
the midpoint of the intervention and at the conclusion of the intervention
– might serve as useful dependent variables.

PSYCHOSOCIAL CONTEXT

The published studies of elective mutism do not address the healthy
manifestations of silence. The background on healthy silence user roles is
missing and with it the wider meaning of speech refusal. Unanswered is
the question: "What are the functions of silence in human communication?"
The majority of the interpretations of elective mutism favor a reinforcement
paradigm. The human experience of silence is undoubtedly more complex
than what can be portrayed in an antecedent-response-consequence
model. The reinforcement model seems to discount the importance of the
experience of silence. An operant conditioning paradigm is useful for
explaining the maintenance of speech refusal but the paradigm is not
adequate for addressing the acquisition of the mutistic response. Rarely
do studies report asking clients why they elected to be "silence users."
The number of investigations which report asking clients these or similar
questions can be counted on the fingers of one hand.
    Western cultures place speaking on a higher plane than listening. Psychic
pain sometimes creates the condition of silence which is a prerequisite
to the type of self-reflection which may produce, as one end product, a
cessation of the pain. I sometimes ask the question: "Are you listening?"
and I often receive a paraphrase of what I have said. Then I tell the person
that I meant "Are you listening to what you have just said?" – "*Are you
listening to yourself?*" This statement sometimes creates the silence required
for the person to self-reflect. My book is intended to include critiques and
personal reflections which may be useful to persons interested in applied
research and theoretical psychology.
    I can identify people who do engage in the productive use of silence. One

important example is the poet who, through silence, is able to crystallize into words the moments that count. The artist and photographer also capture important images during moments of silence. But with these important exceptions, the usual response is to devalue silence and listening. One only has to be silent for a few moments before one hears people ask, "What's wrong?" Immediately, the silence user is put on the defensive. Rarely are silence users asked to identify what the silence is saying to them, to draw the imagery of the silence, to show what the silence would look like in dance or movement, or to reveal the music or poetry of the silence.

Researchers also need to study the nonverbal communication of silence users in settings in which they speak as well as in contexts in which they elect to be silent. Can we identify differences in the non-verbal communication of silence users in talking and non-talking settings? The behavior profiles of electively mute persons, for example, should include eye contact or its opposite, gaze avoidance. The profile should also include the degree to which electively mute persons encourage or deny communication by assessing the bounds of physical proximity that they will permit in the context of social and personal space. The intriguing observation that electively mute persons may choose to be *physically present* in settings in which they elect to be *verbally absent* also needs to be studied.

CONTINUUM OF INTERVENTIONS

In the part of the book dealing with interventions, I have discussed the generic characteristics of specific techniques. The purpose of the chapters dealing with the interventions for elective mutism is to provide an overview of the foundations of specific interventions which have been applied to elective mutism. There is a logic to the sequence in which the treatments are presented. I have attempted to sequence the treatments according to the continuum of procedures recommended by Brazier and MacDonald (1981). Their recommendation coincides with the principles of normalization. Applied to treatment, this means that the least restrictive and least aversive treatments should be attempted before more restrictive and more aversive procedures are applied. There is little evidence, however, of a recognition of the continuum of procedures in the elective mutism literature. Although educators of exceptional children and youth are well versed in the concept of the least restrictive environment, the awareness has yet to make its appearance in remediation programs for learning and behavior problems. Normalization has wider applications than the physical and social integration of special needs persons into the school and community. One only has to observe the overuse and misuse of the behavior modification procedure of time out to note that the least restrictive environment notion inherent in physical and social integration is not matched by the application of less restrictive treatments.

SYNTHESIS AND INTERPRETATION

There is a need to work toward a synthesis of the findings in the published literature. What is required is a synthesis and clarification of the existing data rather than collecting more data on the same issues. Case studies and small group investigations on elective mutism continue to be published. There is, however, an unfortunate tendency to collect data at the expense of carefully interpreting the existing data. One important exception is the excellent work by Paniagua and Saeed (1988) which identified the condition of progressive mutism on the basis of critically examining the published reports of atypical mutism. The work of Paniagua and Saeed is in contrast to a research orientation which goes little beyond charting of the data.

I can identify five major purposes of my book which are based on the preceding rationale:
• to provide a background for the behavior problem of elective mutism by identifying healthy users of silence in communication.
• to provide a compendium of practical approaches for assessing and treating elective mutism.
• to suggest etiological models of elective mutism, based on the evaluation and synthesis of case study data.
• to identify recurring themes and major issues in the published literature.
• to identify research questions relating to the assessment and treatment of elective mutism.
I have elected to take the risks involved in constructive interpretation and conceptualization. I hope that my reflections will lead to better ones through the contributions of my readers.

St. John's   Norman Hadley, Ph.D.
Newfoundland   CET, C. Psychol., AFBPsS
Canada

NOTE

[1] I have been guided by the advice of Light and Pillemer (cited in Bausell, 1991) who stressed that (1) "Any reviewing strategy must come from precise questions driving the research"; (2) "disagreements among findings are valuable and should be exploited"; (3) "both numerical and qualitative information play key roles in a good synthesis"; and (4) "statistical precision cannot substitute for conceptual clarity" (p. 4).

ACKNOWLEDGEMENTS

It is a pleasure to acknowledge my indebtedness to the persons who contributed to the development of this book.

A special word of appreciation for typing the numerous revisions of the manuscript: *Ms. Debbie Connors* and *Ms. Jean Claeys*.

For their encouragement and patience: *Nicola Berridge, Evelien Bakker, Tonny van Eekelen, Ellen Girmscheid,* and, especially, *Peter de Liefde,* Editor Humanities and Social Sciences Division of Kluwer Academic Publishers.

For the Foreword: *Dr. Wayne C. Nesbit.*

For sharing their ideas and concerns: *Mr. Ralph Leck, Ms. Heather Higgins* and *Mr. Donald Stevenson.*

For their administrative support during the writing of this book: *Dr. Bernard MacDonald, Dr. Patricia Canning, Dr. Glenn Sheppard, Professor Woody Hewett, Dr. Clifford Carbno, Dean Robert Crocker, Dean Robin Enns* and *Dr. Shaun McNiff.*

For the opportunity to complete the manuscript in my native Nova Scotia: *Dr. Bernard MacDonald, Dr. James Muir* and *The Nova Scotia Teachers College.*

For the illustrations: *Mr. Jerry Porter.*

For assistance with the revisions in the month prior to the deadline: *Mrs. Carolyn Lono* and *Ms. Janice Neary.*

For permission to quote and summarize:
Table 2.1 from *Psycholinguistic: Experiments in Spontaneous Speech* (p. 14) by F. Goldman Eisler, 1968, New York: Academic Press. Copyright 1968.
Note 8.1 from Children and Deception by K.M. Quinn (pp. 115–117) in R. Rogers (ed.) *Clinical Assessment of Malingering and Deception,* 1988, New York: Guilford Press. Copyright 1988.

Tables 12.1, 12.2 and 12.3 from *Listening to Children Talking* (pp. 40, 41, 42, respectively) by J. Tough, 1985, London: Ward Lock Educational. Copyright 1985.

Figure 19.1 from brochure of Voicelite by Behavioral Controls Inc., 3818 West Mitchell Street, Milwaukee, WI 53215, USA or fax 1-414-671-3332.

CHAPTER 1

ELECTIVE MUTISM: NATURE AND CHARACTERISTICS

HISTORICAL INTRODUCTION

Spieler (cited in Salfield, 1950) identified three major types of psychogenic mutism: hysterical mutism, elective mutism and idiogenic mutism. Schizophrenic mutism, a fourth type, was added by Salfield (1950). Mutism may occur in schizophrenia but it is accompanied by withdrawal, lack of affect, catatonic features, and deterioration in habits. Hysterical mutism is the unconscious expression of an emotional problem in a physical symptom. In this case, the problem is expressed in mutism. In hysterical, and even in schizophrenic mutism, children have surprised their parents by speaking in emergency situations. Idiogenic mutism is a rare condition in which the patient imagines that the speech organs are diseased.

Table 1.1 presents excerpts from the DSM–III–R diagnostic criteria and the recommended guidelines for DSM–IV as proposed in the publication *DSM–IV Options: Work in Progress* (1991). DSM–III–R places elective mutism within the category encompassing "Disorders Usually First Evident in Infancy, Childhood or Adolescence." *DSM–IV Options: Work in Progress* proposes to include this disorder in the "Speech and Language Disorders" section because elective mutism involves a disorder in communication. A second option is to place elective mutism in the section which covers "Anxiety Disorders of Childhood or Adolescence [because] many children with Elective Mutism have anxiety as an associated feature or have an accompanying Anxiety Disorder" (p. 34). We shall have to wait, however, for the publication of DSM–IV to see how the issue is resolved.

RELUCTANT SPEECH

A distinction can be made between elective mutism, which implies an absence of speech in the target situation, and reluctant speech, which is described as low-incidence speech in the target situation (Brown and Doll, 1988). Williamson *et al.* (1977) have noted that certain cases of speech refusal are not as persistent and continuous as typical cases of elective mutism. Rather than being characterized by a complete absence of speech, as is the case with elective mutism, persons exhibiting reluctant speech display occasional verbal behaviors when prompted in social situations other than the home environment (Morin *et al.*, 1982). A number of cases of

Table 1.1. Diagnostic guidelines for elective mutism.

American psychiatric association

DSM–III–R	DSM–IV OPTIONS
A. Persistent refusal to talk in one or more social situations (including at school).	A. Persistent refusal to talk in one or more social situations (such as in school) in children with demonstrated ability to speak.
B. Ability to comprehend spoken language and speak.	B. The disturbance interferes with educational and/or occupational achievement, or with social communication.
	C. Mutism is not due to a lack of fluency in the language required by the social situation [e.g., recent immigrant children who may be mute in school before learning English] and is not due to embarrassment about having a speech or language disorder (e.g., stuttering).
	D. Duration[1] of at least one month (not limited to the first month of school).

[1] DSM–III–R indicated no duration; ICD–10 requires six months but this might unnecessarily delay treatment.

reluctant speech have been reported in the literature (Straughan *et al.*, 1965; Williamson *et al.*, 1977; Morin *et al.*, 1982). Subak *et al.* (1982) also distinguish between spontaneous speech which is self-initiated and speech elicited by requests which they term responsive.

ELECTIVE MUTISM

"Like a camera, the silent patient sees, hears, records, and retains everything, but does not respond verbally." (Subak *et al.*, 1982, p. 335). Chethik (1973) used the term "silence users" to mean speech refusal. Other synonyms found in the literature include voluntary mutism, voluntary silence, elective mutism and selective mutism (Louden, 1987). Elson *et al.* (1965) defined elective mutism as a selective refusal to speak that can occur in children with average intelligence without neurological impairment and which first is observed when the child is separated from the family, usually at the time of entering kindergarten. These authors also claimed that elective mutism is sometimes accompanied by school refusal such as school phobia.

An exclusion definition was offered by Friedman and Karagan (1973). Their definition identified the absence of: (1) a physical defect of the speech mechanism, (2) a speech and language disorder, (3) mental defect and (4) evidence of physical or psychological trauma. Like other writers, they also asserted that the electively mute individual elected to speak to selected persons in certain surroundings. A definition by exclusion is not entirely satisfactory, however, because one or more of the above problems may precede or accompany elective mutism. According to Bauermeister and Jemail (1975), elective mutism may be defined as:

A particular verbal behavior problem in which fully developed speech is emitted in the presence of some persons but suppressed in the presence of others (p. 246).

For Wulbert et al. (1973) an electively mute individual was conceptualized as:

A person who will speak only in restricted stimulus settings. Usually, an electively mute child will exhibit adequate verbal behavior with its family in the home setting but will remain silent in the presence of other persons outside the home. Stimulus control refers to the extent to which the presence or absence of a stimulus controls the probability of a response. For electively mute children, verbal behavior is under the strong stimulus control of their parents and family (p. 435).

Kehle et al. (1990) describe elective mutism as speech refusal that is "dependent on clear situational boundaries." These authors provide one of the clearest definitions. They described electively mute children as "children who do not verbally respond in self-selected situations." By definition, the term excludes mutism secondary to problems of organicism (aphasia, hearing difficulties or dysarthrias) mental deficiency or disorders of thought process (Subak et al., 1982).

SYMPTOM FUNCTIONS OF ELECTIVE MUTISM

Carr and Afnan (1989) claimed that the elective mutism of their female client served multiple functions: (1) Mutism permitted the young female client to express her anger at those who attempted to seize her position as "the baby" in her social network without suffering reprisals, (2) it helped the client to reduce anxiety about separation and entry into new relationships, (3) the symptom served a useful function for the parent. The elective mutism of a child may provide the parent with a way of legitimizing his or her over-involved relationship with the client and (4) elective mutism may permit teachers and other adults to legitimize their response of socializing the child into an invalid role.

Clinicians need to be very cautious in treating mutism in children. According to Shreeve (1991) elective mutism may be an unspoken complaint of severe depression. In other words, elective mutism may be a way that the child "masks" his or her depression.

CHILDHOOD AND ADOLESCENT ELECTIVE MUTISM

Based on their investigation of two silent adolescent girls, Kaplan and Escoll (1973) observed a number of features which they claimed distinguish between childhood and adolescent elective mutism. Table 1.2, adapted from Kaplan and Escoll's study, presents the major distinctions:

Table 1.2. Child and adolescent elective mutism.

Characteristic	Childhood elective mutism	Adolescent elective mutism
Onset	Before age 6	After age 12
Partial mutism	Peers, strangers and therapist	Peers, family and therapist
Chief complaint	Speech refusal	Problems such as stealing, suicide attempts
Dynamics	Expression of dependency and separation anxiety	Expression of disagreement towards family member(s)

Meijer (1979) argued that electively mute children speak to people outside the family but not to family members because:

The mother feels lonely, deprived, neglected, depressed and resentful towards the father. There are frequent instances of serious quarrels and lack of verbal communication between the parents. The mother ties a highly sensitive young child to her, who then feels entangled in a loyalty conflict with regard to the parents and develops a resulting fear of commitment by verbal communication with other adults. The child's fear of arousing the mother's resentment and of separation from her, increases with the level of its hostile dependency on her. The fear is reduced by the symptom of elective mutism by speaking only to children and some chosen adults who are felt to be outside the parental conflict sphere (p. 93).

Atoynatan (1986) also observed that an electively mute child may comply with the mother by not communicating with family members who are objects of her anger and frustration. By refusing to speak, the electively mute children perceive that they will be protected by the parent to whom they align themselves.

The work of Meijer (1979) and Atoynatan (1986) can readily be linked to Reed's anxiety-reducing elective mutism and manipulative-attention getting elective mutism. Passive aggression expressed through the medium of silence (perhaps directed at the father because of his "neglect" of the mother) and the anxiety-reducing function (not speaking to the father) ensures the continued love and support of the mother. Anxiety-reduction and manipulation are therefore *simultaneously expressed in the act of silence.* However, in contrast to Reed's account of manipulation, the manipulation discussed by Meijer and Atoynatan is initiated by a parent and primarily serves the motivations of the parent.

Browne *et al.* (1963) asserted:

The therapeutic focus remains on the child and treatment consists of doing things with him and to him. If therapy of the parents is mentioned it seems to be of an instructional or pedagogic nature (p. 607).

Browne *et al.* also argued that the appropriate unit of diagnosis and treatment is the family. They asserted:

If one makes an intensive study of the entire family, it becomes apparent that the symptom in these children represents not only individual psychopathology, but family psychopathology (p. 607).

Although stressing the potential contribution of the family to elective mutism they were reluctant to include the specific contributions of a disturbed family in their discussion of elective mutism. Browne *et al.*'s (1963) reference to the earlier work of Adams and Glasser (1954), however, seems to indicate that they were ambivalent about the role of family psychopathology in the diagnosis of elective mutism. They concluded that Adams and Glasser:

. . . included some cases which we would have excluded by definition. They particularly emphasized that the children in their cases came from severely disturbed home situations (p. 607).

PROGRESSIVE MUTISM

Based on a careful review of several cases of atypical elective mutism, Panigua and Saeed (1987) described a type of mutism which does not correspond to elective mutism. The name they gave to this type of mutism was "progressive mutism." According to Panigua and Saeed, the concept of progressive mutism includes all of the diagnostic criteria for elective mutism with the exception that the child does not talk to anyone, including family members and close friends. Table 1.3 summarizes the data on which they developed their argument for progressive mutism.

Table 1.3. Rationale for progressive mutism.

Research study	Clinical case details
Panigua & Saeed (1987)	Verbal communication before age 5 with progressive decrease in verbal behavior to parents and others to near-zero frequency.
Chethik (1973)	Near-zero verbal interactions with parents and zero communication to friends in school, and adults and relatives at home and in school.
Straughton (1968)	Infrequently spoke to close friends.
Reed (1963)	Near-zero communication with parents.

CHAPTER 2

PSYCHOSOCIAL FACTORS OF SILENCE

GRAMMATICAL PAUSES

Silences are as much a part of speech as vocal utterances. Each sequence in spoken communication is characterized by consecutive sound-silence segments. Common grammatical silences may include:
- "Natural" punctuation points, e.g. the end of a sentence.
- Immediately preceding a conjunction whether (i) co-ordinating, e.g., and, but, neither, therefore, or (ii) subordinating, e.g., if, when, while, as, because.
- Before relative and interrogative pronouns, e.g., who, which, what, why, whose.
- When a question is indirect or implied, e.g., "I don't know whether I will."
- Before all adverbial clauses of time (when), manner (how) and place (where).
- When complete parenthetical references are made, e.g., "You can tell that the words – this is the phonetician speaking – the words are not sincere" (Goldman Eisler, 1968, p. 13).

NON-GRAMMATICAL PAUSES

There are also silences which do not facilitate communication and may even impede communication. These are called non-grammatical pauses and include:
- Where a gap occurs in the middle or at the end of a phrase, e.g. "In each of // the cells of the body // . . ."
- Where a gap occurs between words and phrases repeated, e.g., (i) "The question of the // of the economy." (ii) "This attitude is narrower than that // than that of many South Africans."
- Where a gap occurs in the middle of a verbal compound, e.g. "We have // taken issue with them and they are // resolved to oppose us."
- Where the structure of a sentence was disrupted by a [reconsideration] or a false start, e.g., "I think the problem of de Gaulle is the // what we have to remember about France is . . ." (Goldman Eisler, 1968, p. 13).

6

DECISION-MAKING SILENCES

There are a number of decision points which are marked by silences in verbal communication. These include semantic choices (content decisions), syntactic choices (word sequencing decisions) and lexical choices associated with selecting words to fit the syntactic plan and the content. All three decisions may delay the production of speech (Goldman Eisler, 1968).

In Goldman Eisler's research, subjects were shown cartoons with no verbal captions. They were asked to describe the content of the story depicted in the pictures and conclude by formulating the meaning or moral of the story. The cartoons were not removed during the story-telling so memory was not a significant factor. Goldman Eisler (1968) reported the following measurements:

- Period of intake (taken from "Got it" to its last word).
- Initial delay of description (period from "Got it" to words of description).
- Duration of description (taken from "Got it" to its last word).
- Duration of interpretation (starting from the last word of description and taken to the last word of the interpretation).
- Length of pauses in descriptions.
- Length of pauses in interpretation.
- Number of words in description.
- Number of words in interpretation (p. 54).

Goldman Eisler's research revealed that: (1) the rate of speech production was greater for description of cartoons than for interpretation of the meaning of the cartoons, (2) the rate of speech for both description and interpretation of cartoons increased after repeatedly responding to the same cartoons and (3) hesitation pauses within sentences was a function of the predictability of the words following the pauses. A summary of the findings of the study are found in Table 2.1.

There are several hypotheses which account for filled and unfilled pauses ("ahs" and similar expressions), see Table 2.2. Hypothesis 1, exemplified by the work of Mahl (1956), is that high anxiety arousal increases the frequency and duration of silent pauses. The work of Pope *et al.* (1970), Siegman (1978a), and Siegman (1978b) represents Hypothesis 2 – that anxiety arousal increases speech and reduces the frequency and duration of silent pauses. Hypothesis 3 is illustrated by the seminal work of Goldman Eisler (1968). She argued that silent pausing reflects the cognitive processes that are occurring during the pauses.

Goldman Eisler (1968) found that cartoon interpretations were associated with longer silent pauses than interpretations, a finding which she attributed to the more complex level of information processing that is required of the subject in the interpretation task than in the description task. Descriptions were associated with significantly higher silent-pause

Table 2.1. Distributions of pause durations for different samples of spontaneous speech.

Speech situations	Less than 0.5 seconds	1.0 seconds	2.0 seconds	3.0 seconds	3.0–8.0 seconds	8.0 seconds and over
	Percentage occurrence (means) of pauses of different duration					
Cartoon descriptions (spontaneous)	47.8	23.7	17.2	6.0	4.6	0.7
Cartoon interpretation (spontaneous)	43.6	19.8	16.3	8.8	9.6	1.9
Cartoon descriptions (learned)	59.6	24.3	12.7	2.7	0.7	0.0
Cartoon interpretation (learned)	63.7	20.0	13.5	2.0	0.8	0.0
Discussions (adults)	49.9	37.1	12.0	1.0	0.0	0.0
Discussions (adolescents)	41.4	41.1	16.0	1.3	0.1	0.0
Psychiatric interviews	16.4	33.9	28.6	10.8	9.6	0.6

Note: From *Psycholinguistics: Experiments in Spontaneous Speech* (p. 14) by F. Goldman Eisler, 1968, New York: Academic Press. Copyright 1968. Adapted with permission.

Table 2.2. Hypotheses to account for filled and unfilled pauses.

Hypothesis 1 Anxiety arousal ↓ Silence (↑)	Hypothesis 2 Anxiety arousal ↓ Silence (↓)	Hypothesis 3 Decision making ↑ Silence (↑)

ratios (but not filled pause such as "ahs" and similar expressions) than the interpretations.

The evidence favors the decision-making hypothesis although each of the three hypotheses may apply in specific cases. Furthermore, task instructions influence the duration of hesitation pauses. Goldman Eisler (1968) indicates that requests to concisely respond are correlated with increases in silent or unfilled hesitation pauses. Siegman (1979) attributed the inverse relation between conciseness and fluency to the fact that the respondents not only had to interpret the cartoons, but, in addition, they had to concisely express their interpretations. This two-fold requirement introduced additional difficulty into the task and therefore the respondents required additional time to formulate their answers. Therefore, there was an increase in hesitation pauses. Siegman (1979) concluded that "the critical 'mediating variable' may be task difficulty which influences both productivity and fluency, rather than conciseness per se" (Siegman, 1979, p. 155).

RATE OF SPEECH PRODUCTION

Frequency is a useful method of computing the rate of speech production; the basic formula for computing frequency is *Number ÷ Time*. The targets for determining the rate of speech production are the number of sounds or words divided by the observation time. The rate of speech production depends on the number and duration of silences which occur during the utterance time. The rate is influenced by the number and duration of grammatical silences and non-grammatical silences such as planning of utterances and breath intakes during speech respectively. Goldman Eisler (1968) found that the ceiling for speech articulation was between 4.4–5.9 syllables per second.

SILENCE-SPEECH RATIO

Practitioners and applied researchers are frequently interested in determining the relative proportion of silences and speech during specified observation periods. The speech-silence ratio is computed by the formula *duration of silence ÷ duration of speech*. There are complicated ways of collecting data for computing speech-silence ratios, but direct observation using a stop watch, which provides a cumulative record of elapsed time, is sufficiently accurate for determining speech-silence ratios for the verbal production of electively mute persons.

Discussion

I have found the silence-speech ratio to be a useful measure of the target behavior of electively mute persons. The particular approach that I use is to select several students of the same sex and age as the electively mute students and randomly choose one of these students to serve as a "typical child." If we use the "typical child" as a quasi-experimental control it is advisable to collect speech-silence data from him or her at the *same time and in the same setting* that we collect data from the client, that is, during his or her baseline and intervention. The validity of comparing the utterances of the silence user with that of the "typical child" is increased if the speech/silence data is obtained from the same setting for the "typical child" and the silence user. In other words, I record the duration of silences and speech episodes of the "typical child" in the same setting in which the client elects to be silent.

I also compute a speech-silence ratio for the client which is based on an audiotape of a dialogue from a setting in which he or she speaks, such as at home with family members. I owe the success of this approach to

the cooperation of parents in unobtrusively taping a number of conversations in which their child was a participant. The speech-silence ratio for
the "typical case," obtained from the setting in which the electively mute
individual does not talk, and the speech-silence ratio of the electively mute
person, based on a setting in which he or she does talk, yields useful information for establishing treatment expectations. *In addition to providing
useful assessment information about the pattern of silences used by the
client, the speech-silence ratio is also a useful dependent variable for
monitoring intervention effects. Speech-silence ratios can be readily charted
and this facilitates making intra-individual comparisons between baseline
and treatment.*

CONVERSATIONAL RHYTHMS

During a dialogue, vocal activity switches from one speaker to another.
An utterance is characterized by all of the speech of the active speaker
until the inactive speaker begins to speak (see arrows showing speaker
switches in Fig. 2.1). Jaffe and Feldstein (1970) observed that vocalizations may be concurrent with, or independent of gestural activity.

One of the clearest descriptions of the parameters of the Jaffe and
Feldstein model is provided by Dabbs, Ruback and Evans (1987). They
asserted that:

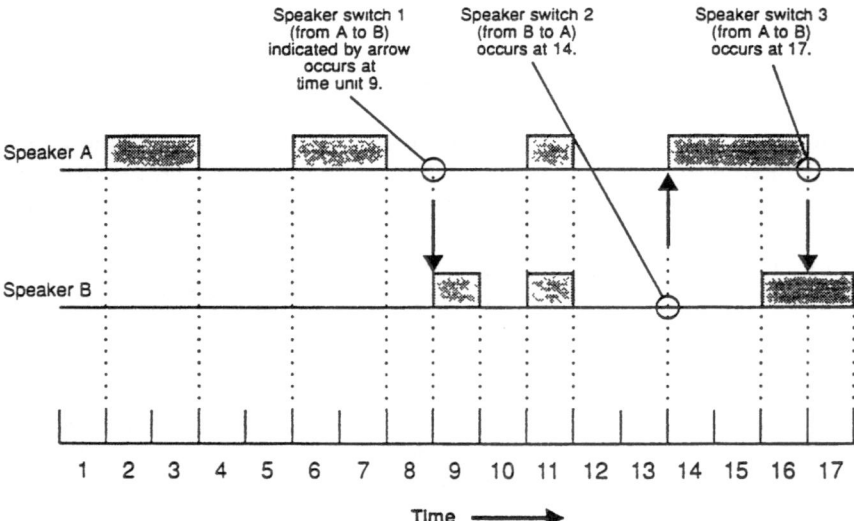

Fig. 2.1. Temporal rhythm in sample dyadic conversation schematized according to the
Jaffe and Feldstein Procedures.

The basic parameter in the Jaffe and Feldstein scheme is the individual *turn*, which is made up of a speaker's vocalizations and pauses. Silence that ends a turn is a *switching pause*, and it is always followed by the beginning of the other speaker's turn. When one speaker has the turn and is speaking and the other joins in, this speech on the part of the second speaker is called *simultaneous speech; interruptive simultaneous speech leads to a change of turn, and noninterruptive speech* does not (p. 503).

An utterance is a stimulus for the inactive speaker's subsequent utterance. The end of the active speaker's utterance and the beginning of the inactive speaker's utterance are marked by a brief silence. We might view this as the time it takes the inactive speaker to respond. The reaction time may be positive or negative. The reaction time is positive if the inactive speaker begins to talk *after* the active speaker has completed an utterance. Consequently, forward timing is involved because timing begins from the end of the active speaker's utterance until the inactive speaker begins to talk.

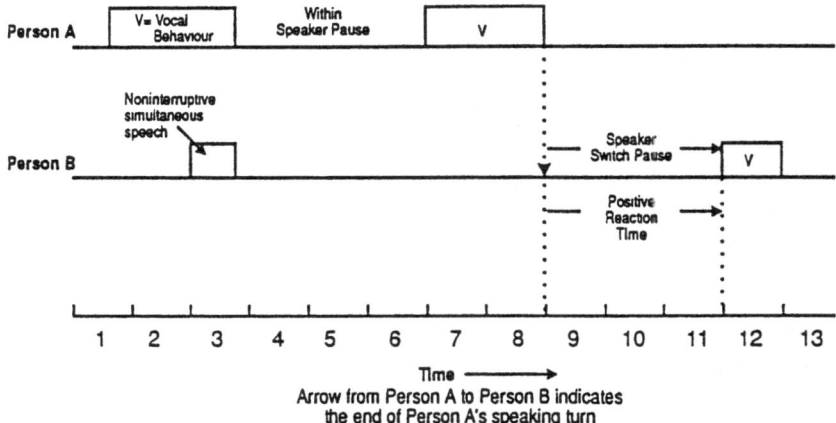

Fig. 2.2. Positive reaction time involving forward timing schematized according to the Jaffe and Feldstein Procedure.

The reaction time is negative if the inactive speaker begins to talk *before* the active speaker has completed his or her utterance. A negative reaction time involves backward timing from when the active speaker stopped talking to the beginning of speech by the other participant. A negative reaction time[1] between speaking turns indicates that the two individuals are speaking at the same time and therefore qualifies as simultaneous speech – and either an intrusive or non-intrusive interruption.

Silences ordinarily occur at the end of utterances but they may also occur during the speech of the active speaker (Jaffe and Feldstein, 1970). One-way dialogue is the norm in human communication and this means that

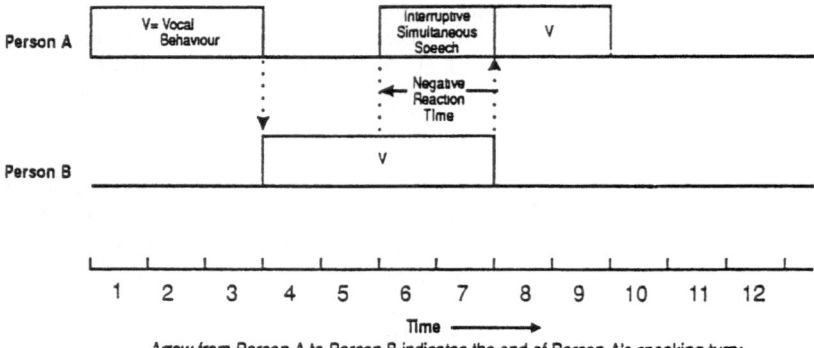

Arrow from Person A to Person B indicates the end of Person A's speaking turn;
arrow from Person B to Person A shows the end of B's speaking turn

Fig. 2.3. Negative reaction time involving backward timing schematized according to the Jaffe and Feldstein Procedure.

simultaneous speech is a violation of speaking patterns in conversations. In a monologue, an active speaker holds the floor continuously and the speech contains intra-speaker pauses, but not switching pauses or simultaneous speech (See Fig. 2.4). Intra-speaker pauses do not result in speaker switches. There are, however, exceptions which require synchrony of vocal activity such as choral singing and cheering. In a monologue the listener may complain of the lack of speaker-switches which is characteristic of a dialogue. If a monologue continues for too long, the inactive speaker may have no choice but to talk at the same time as the active speaker. Indeed, the listener must violate the "dysynchrony rule" if he or she is to break the monologue and participate in the conversation.

According to Jaffe and Feldstein (1970) there are four types of turn-endings (See Fig. 2.5). Overlong endings and interruptions violate turn-taking rules. An overlong silence occurs when one person stops talking and another initiates a turn after a silence greater than 2.9 seconds. An interruption is a turn-ending resulting from the simultaneous speech of a person not owning the speaking floor. These researchers (Jaffe and Feldstein,

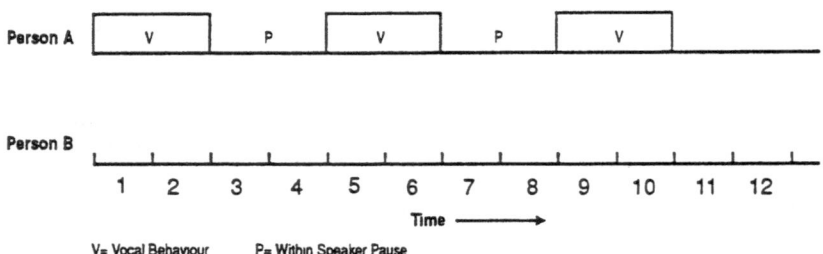

Fig. 2.4. Monologue schematized according to the Jaffe and Feldstein Procedure.

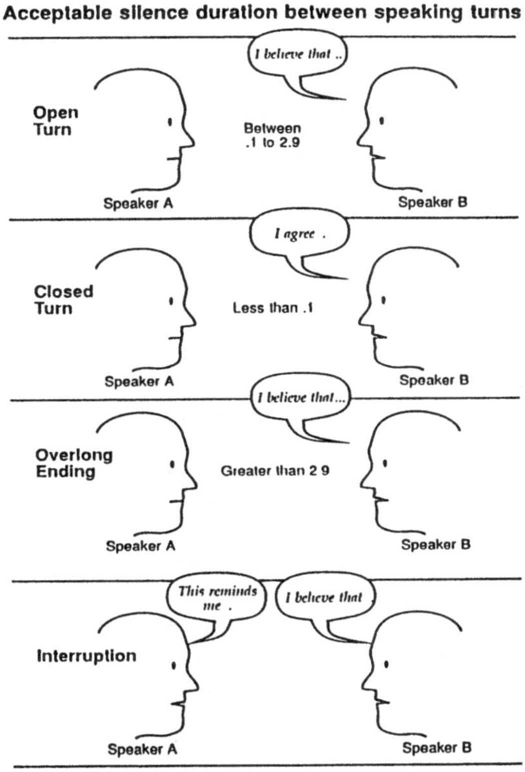

Acceptable silence duration between speaking turns

Fig. 2.5. Turn-endings in diadic conversations.

1970) also identified two types of silences which are within the "range of comfort" for turn-taking. These are open-turns in which a person initiates a turn after .1 second to 2.9 seconds of silence and a closed turn in which the person begins to speak after .1 second or less of silence after the other participant stops talking.

TURN-TAKING IN GROUP CONVERSATIONS

Dabbs *et al.* (1987) claim that the Jaffe and Feldstein model does not address sounds and silences in group conversations involving three or more participants. They, therefore, argued that:

In groups larger than dyads a turn-taker may fall silent while several others are speaking at once, in which case there is no obvious way to decide who has the turn. No new turn-taker has emerged (no one else is speaking alone), but it hardly seems appropriate to continue crediting the turn to the original speaker, who is now silent while others are speaking. Another problem with using the concept of alternating individual turns in groups arises when there is silence for a moment following a speaker, and then two or more speakers begin at once. The Grouptalk model proposes the notion of *group turn* to cover these contingencies.

A group turn begins when an individual turn-taker has fallen silent and two or more other persons are speaking. The other persons may have interrupted the original turn-taker, or they may simultaneously have begun to speak following a silence. The group turn ends the instant an individual again speaks alone. Analogously to individual turns, group turns may contain *group vocalizations* and *group pauses* and end with *group-switching pauses*. During a group turn the set of people who are speaking together may vary, but no one will be speaking alone (p. 504).

Discussion

I have discussed both the Jaffe and Feldstein dyadic model and the Dabbs *et al.* "Grouptalk" model because both contexts are relevant for human conversation. Dialogue involving trusted friends and acquaintances often takes the form of two-person conversations. Our verbal interactions, however, are not limited to one-to-one conversations. We may be invited to speak to a group but even in this context there is the opportunity for dialogue. We participate in group conversations both inside and outside the home. We discuss our views, disclose our feelings and pain, present our arguments in favour of our own or another's stance, offer suggestions and elaborate on the statements of other members. The Dabbs *et al.* (1989) "grouptalk" scheme is important for the study of electively mute behavior because (1) a group context is more often than not the setting in which the person elects to be silent and (2) in the majority of interventions, the exposure of the electively mute person to speaking in a group setting begins with exposure to two-person groups and then to groups which are successively larger than two people.

VISUAL BEHAVIOR IN TURN-TAKING

We have primarily discussed the role of speaker-switch silences, intraspeaker silences and simultaneous speech including intrusive and non-intrusive interruptions. These parameters dealt with cues modulated within the auditory modality. There is evidence, however, that visual behavior can serve a regulatory function in conversational turn-taking. Kendon's (1967) research and analyses indicates that a prolonged gaze at the end of an utterance functions as a turn-yielding signal. Averting a gaze during a conversation is an attempt to reduce distracting visual signals emitted by the conversational parties. Kendon's position, however, has not gone unchallenged. Beattie (1981), for example, reported that prolonged gazes in dyadic conversations delay rather than produce immediate turn-taking. Furthermore, this researcher argued that when visual feedback is reduced or eliminated an increase in interruptions may be observed to occur, and verbal cues may play a greater role in assigning speaking turns. A factor which may impact on an individual's emitting prolonged gazes is the status of the participants. Kalma (1992) studied prolonged gazes between high and low status persons in simulated employer-applicants contexts. He found that the employers (the appointed high status persons) displayed prolonged gazes significantly more than the interviewees (the appointed low status individuals).

DISCUSSION

We know very little about the electively mute person's handling of conversational turn-taking. Yet, information about a person's switch-pauses, intra-speaker pauses and simultaneous speech (interrupting others or being interrupted by others) is relevant for our understanding of elective mutism. What is the speech of the electively mute person like in the settings in which he is observed to talk? Would the observations from settings in which the electively mute person talks indicate that he or she ordinarily responds to speaker-switch silences or other nonverbal turn-taking signals such as eye contact? Indeed, do the observations suggest that he or she recognizes the auditory or visual turn-taking cues? Or, does the electively mute person recognize the turn-taking signals, yet not respond to them?

And what happens when the silence user does speak? Is the person encouraged or discouraged from speaking and what is the form of the encouragement or discouragement? If the reactions of the listeners are primarily negative is it possible that the electively mute person anticipates a similar reaction to his or her verbal presence in other settings – and hence behaves accordingly. In settings in which he or she speaks, does he or she have a habit of talking while the active speaker is talking? Being more specific, do observations indicate that his or her simultaneous speech is typically interruptive, non-interruptive or both? And what is the reaction of the active speaker when he or she hears the person talking at the same time that he or she is talking?

Even information obtained by direct observation or by practitioner-client interviews will yield an incomplete "picture" of the speaking patterns of electively mute individuals. It might be useful, therefore, to determine the impressions of family members concerning the electively mute individual's conversational rhythms? Does the electively mute person respond to identifiable turn-taking signals? Do family members feel that he or she reluctantly participates in conversations? Or, do they suggest that he or she typically dominates conversations? By dominating conversations, I mean the conversational parameters of monologue, non-intrusive interruptions and intrusive interruptions referred to by Jaffe and Feldstein (1970).

Does he or she respond to speaker-switch pauses without having to be verbally prompted? If he or she does respond, does there seem to be inordinately long "speaker-switch" pauses? It is important to note that a "speaker-switch" pause is a stimulus for the inactive speaker to talk – and it is the inactive speaker, therefore, who determines the duration of the silence. Here, we are referring to what might be called "awkward silences." In this case, I speculate that it is the previous speaker – the one who initiated the silence – who experiences the greater discomfort. It is reasonable to expect, however, that the duration of the silence in speaker-switch pauses will vary with the interest of the listener in the active speaker's topic of conversation and/or how familiar the inactive speaker is with the topic. Certainly, we are tempted to consider this argument because it is supported by direct observation and psycholinguistic research (see, for example, Table 2.1).

Inactive speakers have the option of shortening or lengthening speaker-switch pauses. We should therefore attempt to determine the reason for excessively long silences which violate conversational rhythms. This means that we need to be watchful of speaker-switch pauses which are subjectively determined to be excessively long by external observers, initiators of speaker-switch pauses and electively mute persons themselves.

On the basis of clinical experience, however, it seems that if electively mute persons detect switch pauses, they ignore them; if they observe the gazes of the active speaker, they do not respond to the signals by speaking. And, on hearing the verbal prompt – "It's your turn to speak," they still do not respond. This argument is not so far fetched. Those of us who are teachers can recall the way in which our students seem to ignore our silent pause, avert our gaze and refuse to respond to verbal encouragement when we ask the class to respond to a question. On some such occasions, the whole class seems to become electively mute. The lack of verbal contact with us by some of our students perhaps indicates that they do not wish to respond or that they would like to respond but do not respond because they are unsure about what would constitute an appropriate response. *Perhaps if these temporary episodes of "group elective mutism" were explored, they would be found to share many of the characteristics of the elective mutism of individuals. If these arguments are accurate, then, this suggests that elective mutism involves observable non-compliance with the turn-taking cues of switch pauses, visual contact and even verbal prompts.*

If we are going to understand elective mutism we must abandon the molar focus involving "speaking episodes" and take a more molecular approach. The discussion of turn-endings is, therefore, intended to sensitize practitioners to the types of turn endings which may occur during conversations. The self-reports of participants and the impressions of external observers based on samples of conversations of electively mute persons obtained from settings in which they speak would seem to be a useful baseline against which to compare the turn-endings of clients when they began to participate in conversations in formerly non-speaking settings.

The next major section of this chapter addresses gender differences in conversational style. This is important because whether or not speech is judged to be intrusive or non-intrusive depends on the gender of the person who is interrupted and the gender of the person who initiates the interruption. Males appear to differ in their conversational style from that of females – including the interpretation they give to non-intrusive interruptions.

GENDER DIFFERENCES IN CONVERSATIONAL STYLE

Because elective mutism seems to be favored by females, it is important to be aware of the gender differences in conversational style because this may be one of the factors which put females at risk for developing elective mutism. The differences to be discussed are exemplary rather than inclusive but they target differences in conversational style which may be overlooked.

Identifying Interruptions

A frequently used procedure for identifying interruptions is based on the overlap definition. One either observes a conversation or listens to an audio recording of one and records the number of times and/or the duration of time that one hears two voices speaking at the same time. The procedure is accurate, however, only to the extent that it identifies people who are talking at the same time. This means that the number or duration of overlaps is no guarantee, however, that the participants will perceive the overlaps in verbal behavior as intrusive interruptions. I believe that this is because the overlap definition is based on the lowest level of listening which corresponds to the isolation of sounds. Interruptions which are based on the overlap criterion may fail to qualify as an interruption – in the sense of unwanted intrusions – if they are analyzed within the framework of Fessenden's (1966) hierarchy of listening skills. Tannen's interpretation of an excerpt from the research of West and Zimmerman (cited in Tannen, 1990) addresses the issue of intrusive and non-intrusive interventions. (*The vertical lines indicate overlap in the speech of the participants in the following excerpts.*)

FEMALE: So uh you really can't bitch when you've got all those on the same day but I
         uh asked my physics professor if I couldn't chan |ge that|

MALE: |Don't | touch that

FEMALE: What? (pause)

MALE: I've got everything jus'how I want in that notebook, you'll screw it up leafin'
         through it like that (p. 191).

West and Zimmerman consider this an interruption because the second speaker began while
the first speaker was in the middle of a word (change). But considering what was being
said, the first speaker's rights may not have been violated. Although there are other aspects
of this man's talk that make him seem like a conversational bully, interrupting to ask the
woman to stop leafing through his notebook does not in itself violate her right to talk. Many
people, seeing someone handling their property in a way that was destroying their painstaking
organization of it, would feel justified in asking that person to stop immediately, without
allowing further damage to be done while waiting for the appropriate syntactic and
rhetorical moment to take the floor (p. 191).

Support and Elaboration as Interruption

Tannen (1990) claims that "overlaps from high involvement speakers are
cooperative because they do not change the topic but elaborate on it"
(p. 198). Here is an example:

SPEAKER A: I found the clerk very rude; she tried to put me |down and|

SPEAKER B: |I agree; |

            She treats me the same way.

Although Speaker A was not permitted to complete her utterance, the
overlap of Speaker B was clearly supportive of Speaker A. When one
speaker elaborates or agrees while the other person is speaking, it may be
experienced as a non-intrusive interruption rather than as an attempt to seize
an opportunity to speak.

The same verbal response may be viewed differently depending on
whether it is emitted by a male or female. Tannen (1990) reported that
men felt "interrupted by women who overlapped with words of agreement, support and anticipation of how their utterances would end" (p.
210). In other words, men experienced the overlaps as unwanted intrusions. According to Tannen, "elaborating on a different point" *related to the
speaker's topic* does not qualify as a change of topic. A man may, nonetheless, interpret elaborating on a different point from the one he had in mind
as intruding on his right to complete his utterance. This interpretation may
mean that the female is blamed for interrupting when her intention was to
agree with or support the speaker.

Topic Change as Interruption

Murray (1985) claims that an interruption occurs when someone abruptly introduces *a different topic* when the speaker has not made even a single statement.

Here is an example:

SPEAKER A: I |think|

SPEAKER B: |Let |

          Me tell you what happen to me yesterday.

If one person habitually interrupts whenever the other participant in a conversation begins to say something, it violates the right of expression of the other person.

Duration of Speaking Episodes

Women are frequently accused by men of talking too much. The research summarized by Tannen (1990) does not support the view that women talk more than men. In fact, the reverse is true. Men talk more than women especially in public and it seems that men are often silent in the privacy of the home and family. If males are noticeably silent at home, this may create problems if family members view the silences as an uncaring response or as an expression of aloofness. The silence of women is frequently cited as evidence of lack of power in the communication context. At the same time, the refusal to speak by men is often cited as a demonstration of their power.

Differences in Meaning Attributed to Utterances

The meaning attributed to phrases such as "I'm sorry" differs between males and females. The example from Tannen (1990) will show how an apparent apology may have a very different meaning depending on whether a male or female is the recipient of the message:

A teacher was having trouble with a student widely known to be incorrigible. Finally, she sent the boy to the principal's office. Later the principal approached her in the teachers' lounge and told her the student had been suspended. The teacher replied, "I'm sorry," and the principal reassured her, "It's not your fault." The teacher was taken aback by the principal's reassurance, because it had not occurred to her that the student's suspension might be her fault until he said it. To her, "I'm sorry" did not mean "I apologize;" it meant "I'm sorry to hear that." "I'm sorry" was intended to establish a connection to the principal by implying, "I know you must feel bad about this; I do too." She was framing herself as connected to him by similar feelings. By interpreting her words of shared feeling as an apology, the principal introduced the notion that she might be at fault, and framed himself as one-up, in a position to absolve her of guilt (p. 232).

Listening Styles

Males and females have different ways of demonstrating that they are listening. Tannen (1991) discusses these differences and how they may lead to faulty interruptions which negatively impact on communication. Tannen claimed that:

. . . many women complain that their partners don't listen to them. But men make the same complaint about women, although less frequently. The accusation "You're not listening" often really means "You don't understand what I said in the way that I meant it," or "I'm not getting the response I wanted." Being listened to can become a metaphor for being understood and being valued (pp. 141–142).

Matching Problems

Women tend to tell a problem of their own in response to listening to a problem of another person. The intent of this communication is to establish a connection with the speaker. Males, however, may interpret the woman's response as an attempt to discount the importance of their problems. Tannen (1990) claims that:

If women are often frustrated because men do not respond to their troubles by offering matching troubles, men are often frustrated because women do. Some men not only take no comfort in such a response, they take offense. For example, a woman told me that when her companion talks about a personal concern – for example, his feelings about growing older – she responds, "I know how you feel; I feel the same way." To her surprise and chagrin, he gets annoyed; he feels she is trying to take something away from him by denying the uniqueness of his experience (p. 51).

An analysis of conversations is provided by Jennifer Coates (1986). According to Coates when a woman takes her speaking-turn, she frequently begins by acknowledging the previous speaker's contribution. Men, on the other hand, generally do not comment on the previous speaker's statement, but instead, focus on making their point. In mixed conversations, this suggests that women may feel that their contributions are being ignored.

Suggestions

Men often interpret suggestions from women as attempts to control or manipulate them. In contrast, women view suggestions as options which are open rather than closed to negotiations. Even more surprising perhaps is that the way in which males and females attempt to influence others can be observed in the play of children. Sachs (1987), for example, found that boys used commands (e.g., "Give me your arm") in playing doctor while girls tended to preface proposals with "Let's" (e.g., "Let's play doctor"). Goodwin (1990) observed the same pattern among black children. The boys whom she described making slingshots gave each other orders (e.g., "Give me that knife") while the girls who were making rings out of bottlenecks used "Let's" to preface their proposals for action (e.g., "Let's go ask him, do you have any more bottles?"). The black girls in the Goodwin study also used words such as (e.g., "We could . . ." and "Maybe we can . . .") rather than direct orders. Their attempts to influence each other was by *way of suggestions*. The boys, however, used commands which specified a particular action for the listener.

TAG QUESTIONS

Tag questions are another area in which males and females differ in their conversational style. Tag questions are added to the end of statements such as, "She's a nice person, isn't she?" Often a tag question is used for emphasis or to determine if the listener agrees with the speaker. Research such as that of Sachs (1987) shows that even among children, girls use more tag questions than boys. Often tag questions go unnoticed but they can be a source of annoyance if the listener feels that the speaker is repeatedly attempting to force him or her to agree.

MIME: THE UNIVERSAL LANGUAGE OF SILENCE

"Mime has been compared to ordinary acting as poetry is compared to prose. A mime can, with a single gesture, convey a world of thought and emotion, just as a line of poetry can convey what might take a chapter of prose." (Shepard, 1971, pp. 9–10)

For instance, if an actor points to another actor (signifying "you"), and then beckons (signifying "come"), and then points to the ground in front of him (signifying "here"), he is behaving verbally. He is literally acting out words. For him to communicate physically, all he need do is beckon, which tells the "you, come here" story more economically. If an actor wants to communicate to an actress that he loves her, he must neither mouth the words, "I love you," nor would he point to himself ("I"), point to his heart ("love"), point to her ("you"). As a mime, he would communicate his love by the way he looks at her and behaves toward her, not by acting out words. The language of the mime must be universal so that practically anybody on this planet can understand his story. Mouthing the words "I love you" would not be understood in France or China, but a look of love, and behavior and responses with the feeling of love in it would be understood anywhere. (p. 3)

Mimes may make some sounds during their performance. They are encouraged, however, to restrict the sounds to those of objects. The mime may occasionally use words but the gestures should not repeat the words. Shepard (1971) clarifies this requirement:

He should use gesture that goes beyond the word, shows other aspects not included in the words, or which communicates something different from the words, so that the audience will receive the combination, which should be more than either the words or the actions separately. The narration might say "Once there was a little girl . . ." The action has to show what kind of a little girl, what she does, how she behaves and relates to others, what her attitudes are, what her peculiarities are. (p. 9)

According to Shepard (1971), if it is absolutely necessary to use a gesture it should come before the word because gesture has a greater impact than words. In my overview, I shall restrict the discussion of techniques to those of magnification, separation and winding up. The effect of these techniques is to enable people to clearly see what is happening – especially those who may be observing at a distance. In this nonverbal method of communication, "the mime does not spell out an emotion in the air; instead, the mime 'experiences an emotion and magnifies the emotion'" (Shepard, 1971, p. 5). Shepard (1971) had this to say about the technique of separating the beginning and ending for each gesture.

he must complete each gesture before beginning the next one. He must separate his actions, in fact, each part of action. In rehearsal he would, for instance, first raise his arm, then stop, lower his hand to his pocket, stop, put his hand in his pocket, stop, take out a key, stop, bring the key to the keyhole, stop, insert the key in the lock, stop, turn it, stop, open the door, stop, and so on. He practices his actions this way, with sharp clear movements, strong impulses, and square corners. In performance, he rounds out the corners, smooths out the actions so that the stops are not really noticeable, but they are, in some subtle way, still there. (p. 5)

In the silent technique of mime, winding up means, for example, that:

before making a downward gesture, he would first move his arm in the opposite direction a bit, thereby making the downward gesture bigger, and more easily seen. Before reaching forward, he would bring his arm back a bit, then forward. Winding up makes for bigger movement, and thereby greater communication, and it also provides a more flowing, more graceful gesture, which is more beautiful to watch; and while our main concern is communication, we do not dismiss beauty. (p. 5)

DISCUSSION

Men and women use interruptions for different purposes. Women interrupt during a speaking turn of another person to give enthusiastic remarks or to indicate that they are actively listening. These types of interruptions, however, are not intended to stop a speaker from completing a turn. Instead, they are an attempt of the inactive speaker to make a connection with the active speaker. In contrast, men's interruptions are frequently used to deny the current speaker's right to complete a turn. The outcome is that in mixed conversations, men's use of interruptions may prevent or delay women from taking a speaking turn. Research into the extent to which intrusive interruptions occur in the conversations of electively mute persons would be a valuable contribution in producing a clearer picture of the conversations of electively mute persons.

NOTE

[1] In Fig. 2.3, Person B is speaking during time units 4–7 inclusive. Speaker B did not stop talking until time unit 7, yet Speaker A (according to the dysynchrony principle, the inactive speaker) started talking at time unit 6 and continued speaking until the end of time unit 9. Speaker A started talking while Speaker B was talking and Speaker B stopped talking at time unit 7. By reading directly from Fig. 2.3 one observes a negative reaction time of 2 time units of interruptive simultaneous speech during units 6 and 7. The speech of Person A is termed interruptive simultaneous speech (ISS) during time units 6 and 7 because the interruption produced a speaker-switch.

CHAPTER 3

COMMUNICATION AND ELECTIVE MUTISM

Applied to elective mutism, the meaning of a silence could lie in the sender, the message, the verbal channel or the receiver. The *sender* could conceal worries about an upcoming event by electing to be *silent*. The silence might also relate to the *message* so that silence is used to control unacceptable hostile impulses. The sender could elect *silence* in the *verbal channel* because of embarrassment about the sound of his voice, accent or speech impediment.

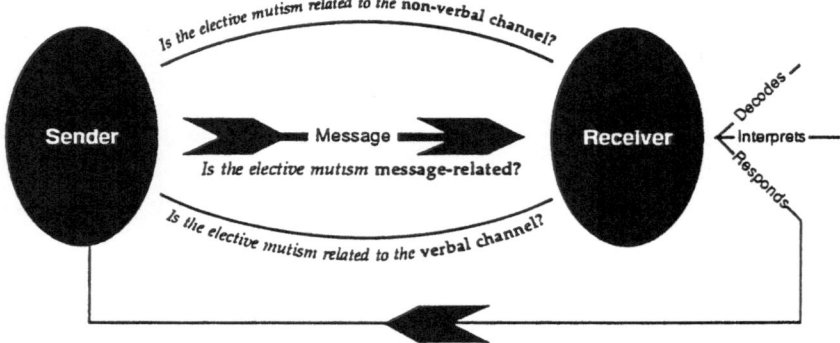

Note: Fig. 3.1 is based on Berko, D.K. (1960). *The Process of Communication.* San Francisco: Rinehart Press.

Fig. 3.1. The communication process and elective mutism.

The *silence* might also be explained by the real or anticipated consequences from the *receiver*. If, for example, the feedback is consistently negative the individual will probably consider the option of using *silence* in the presence of the other person.

The importance of the communication model for understanding and treating elective mutism is supported by Albert-Stewart (1986). He claimed that the major goal of treatment is reducing or eradicating the communication deficits observed in electively mute children.

SYNONYMS OF SILENCE

There are four words which describe variations in silent behavior. The word *taciturn* applies to a person who is habitually uncommunicative. A *reserved* person implies a habitual disposition to be withdrawn in speech and self-restrained in manner. The word *reticent* implies a disinclination to express one's feelings or impart information. The *secretive* person is one who conceals things unnecessarily.

LANGUAGE DEVELOPMENT

The appearance of elective mutism often coincides with the child's first major move out of the family. Krolian (1988) indicates that *the actual level of language development among electively mute children* needs to be studied. Krolian bases his recommendation on his observations of mothers of electively mute children. In talking with the mothers he observed minimal content and expression of identifiable affects in conversations. Carr and Afnan (1989) reported that the peers of their six-year-old electively mute client communicated by using gestures or by passing notes. At the time of referral, teachers, family and peer groups had accepted the elective mutism and developed ways of accommodating to it.

FUNCTIONS OF CONVERSATION

According to Gordon (1969), there are five functions of conversation. The first function fulfils the need to express attitudes, feelings or ideas. The second function is persuasion; the speaker may attempt to get another person to accept a particular view or to take a particular action. Third, the therapeutic function of conversation involves the expression of ideas and feelings within a professional relationship for the purpose of helping an individual to change patterns of behavior. A fourth function is ritual such as saying "hello" and its main purpose is to acknowledge the presence of a person and to provide security in interpersonal relations. The fifth purpose of conversation is the exchange of information and this is important for the research interview or the diagnostic appraisal.

As the above discussion suggests, silence users are deprived of the advantages of conversation. Because the silence user does not engage in conversation, the absence of verbal dialogue during the initial phases of therapy presents a challenge for the therapist. In treating elective mutism, this means that communication is restricted to a monologue in which the therapist speaks for himself or in the case of game play (Schaefer and Reid, 1986) or play therapy to reflect the nonverbal behavior of the client.

SILENCE OF ANONYMITY AND CONFIDENTIALITY

Patients will hesitate in disclosing personal information to their therapists unless they are assured that the content of their discourse is confidential. The extent to which trust is established in the therapeutic relationship even determines if the client will talk and the specific information which he or she will share with the therapist. Breuer and Freud (1957) asserted that, in their combined roles of scientist and clinician, they were continuously confronted with the issue of confidentiality. In their Preface to *Studies in Hysteria* they argued that many patients would never speak if they knew that their disclosures were likely to be included in the published research of clinicians. Clients may carefully monitor and censure their disclosures even if they are guaranteed anonymity of person, place and time.

Although a rare phenomenon, silence can extend to the refusal of the person to reveal his or her name. Strean (1984) documents the case of an adult male who refused to reveal his name until the eighteenth month of a four-year treatment regimen. Although this patient talked, he refused to give his name because he feared that he would "never get a job" if a future employer found that he was receiving treatment. From Strean's account it is very clear that if the therapist had insisted that the patient reveal his name, he would have discontinued treatment.

Strean's report reminds me of the time one of my student's gave a talk to a junior high class on emotional, physical and sexual abuse. The student left her telephone number with the class in case they wanted to contact her. That evening, my student reported that she received a telephone call from an adolescent female who had attended her "talk." The caller refused to reveal her name but revealed that she had attended her talk. The adolescent said that she was being sexually abused by an uncle. The adolescent girl telephoned my student several times over the course of three weeks but still refused to reveal her name.

Upon my suggestion, she reported to Social Services that a junior high school student had contacted her by telephone about being sexually abused. She reported that the young adolescent refused to give her name and that continued contact was dependent on complying with her request. The social worker concurred with the plan of action of my student.

The girl finally agreed to meet my student at a corner restaurant in order to discuss her problem. The adolescent girl still refused to reveal her name but continued to see my student. During the second month of dialogue by telephone and restaurant meetings the adolescent selected one of the options presented by my student – that she go with my student to Social Services in order to plan a course of healing and action. But even here, she agreed to go to Social Services with my student on the condition that she was not required to reveal her name. The sexually abused adolescent was insistent on this requirement. I struggled with the adolescent's request as did my student and the social worker. The social worker agreed to see the young adolescent for one visit without requiring her to give her name.

Shortly after this, the case transferred from my student to the community social worker although the adolescent girl tended to periodically telephone my student. In retrospect, I can only conjecture that had my student insisted that the adolescent girl give her name, she would not have pursued the matter of sexual abuse – at least not with my student at that time.

In spite of the unusual conditions, the young adolescent had contacted the student of her own volition, had agreed to meet with the student of her own volition and had agreed to meet with the social worker of her own volition. On each occasion, the student demonstrated that she had control over how the process evolved and she elected to participate in each of the steps of self-disclosure.

THERAPEUTIC USES OF SILENCE

Barbara (1966), in *The Art of Listening*, describes effective listeners as people who use silence with as much eagerness as they use speech. Listening is often equated with silence but many therapists are not good listeners because they are uncomfortable when they are not speaking. Silence gives the client opportunity to search for words to describe feelings or lived experiences. Finding "the right words" can be therapeutic and allowing the client time to find the words is an effective therapeutic skill (Bradley and Edinberg, 1982).

THERAPISTS' EXPERIENCES OF CLIENTS' SILENCE

Krolian (1988) provides one of the clearest descriptions of the therapist's experience of the silent communication of electively mute children.

They test our very therapeutic mettle by not dealing in the tender of our trade – words. They sit silently in front of you, eyes averted, unmoving and they wait. You may suggest something they'd like to play with but odds are there will be no reply. You may even venture a comment on their sad work, but it will seem to fall on deaf ears. The therapist is left hearing his or her own voice and does not know at first if he or she has been heard, confirmed or denied (pp. 360–361).

In treating electively mute persons, therapists are faced with listening and responding to "word equivalents" which have no sound. Another concern in the treatment of electively mute children is how the therapist negotiates with the client's silence. Krolian (1988) claims that "therapists may be so distressed by the deafening and frustrating silence that . . . they fill the silences themselves thus compromising their empathetic [response] to the child" (p. 361). Krolian also argues that therapists must be aware of the feeling of helplessness and anger elicited by the client's silence and the wish to be the one who succeeds in getting the client to talk.

PRACTITIONERS' RESPONSES TO SILENCE

Murray and Huelskoetter (1991) provide guidelines for dealing with the silent client. They recommend that: (1) therapists should not initiate verbal behavior prematurely because of their own silence-induced anxiety; and (2) therapists should examine the content of the dialogue preceding the silence and observe the nonverbal communication of the client during the silence. Table 3.1 identifies strategies for dealing with selected silences.

Table 3.1. Types of silences and interventions.

Type of silence	Characteristics	Interventions
Blank, empty, blocked	Client says nothing; states, "I have nothing to say." Nonverbal behavior shows anxiety or tension.	Initiate conversaton, perhaps of social nature. Reflect feeling, "It is hard for you to talk now."
Stubborn, resistive	Client feels angry; tries to gain control over another; sets up power struggle.	Avoid reciprocal anger or impatience. Sit in silence; show interest in person. Reflect, "I wonder what is going on within you," or "Tell me your feelings."
Fearful	Client previously intimidated by people when tried to talk; currently intimidated by hallucinations, thoughts or people.	Stay with person; recognize efforts to talk. Be kind and positive. Accept whatever is said. State, "It's OK; you can tell me." Reflect, "It's scary for you to talk," or "You feel afraid?"
Thoughtful	Client resolving difficulties, doing problem solving.	Avoid interrupting thoughts. Suggest, "Share your thoughts with me." Show acceptance.

Note: From *Psychiatric Mental Health Nursing: Giving Emotional Care* by R.B. Murray and M.M.W. Huelskoetter, 1991, Norwalk, CT: Appleton & Lange. Copyright 1991. Reprinted with permission.

Collins (1977) cautions that a client's silence during an interview does not necessarily indicate that he is reflecting on the matter under discussion. Reflection, however, is indicated if the client comments on his own or the therapist's statements which preceded the silence. Reid (1980) presents several options for responding to a client's silence. A therapist can ask about what the client is thinking or feeling, or make a tentative observation related to the client's verbal or gestural responses just prior to the silence. Reid cautions that there is a danger in prolonging the client's discomfort by allowing extended silences. He argues that by prolonging the silence, the therapist might become unnecessarily competitive to see who will be the first to "give in."

PERSISTENT SILENCES

Burton (1972) asserts that "persistent silence without dropping out of therapy, is the most aggressive thing the client can do" (p. 63). Burton suggests that when silence occurs in several consecutive interviews, it is often associated with a history of being punished for talking and sharing information or with controlling or manipulating others by electing to be silent. The therapist's response to client initiated silences should "give the client an opportunity to meet the needs the silence is the cover for" (Burton, 1972, p. 64). According to Burton (1972), a silence should be allowed to continue (1) if the silence is communicating something, (2) serving some function or (3) is not too frightening for the client.

MESSAGES CONVEYED BY THERAPISTS' SILENCE

Spotnitz (1985) claimed that silence can be used by the therapist to communicate three different messages. Motionless silence communicates that the therapist does not wish to disturb the client in any way. He believes that this type of silence is especially appropriate during the early stages of therapy. A second type of silence is shared silence. This silence is characterized by a relaxed body position which is intended to communicate that the therapist is comfortable with the client's and his own silence. A third type, a restless silence, may tactfully convey through behaviors such as coughing that the clinician is eager for the client to talk.

CHAPTER 4

PSYCHOSOCIAL CHARACTERISTICS OF ELECTIVELY MUTE PERSONS PART 1

PHYSICAL HEALTH/ILLNESS

Pustrom and Speers (1964) reported that a child they treated received a skull fracture at nine months as a result of falling out of bed. Later, tonsillitis prevented him from regularly attending school. In the same study, another child underwent herniorrhaphies at eight months and again at two years. One male elective mute in a clinical study by Browne *et al.* (1963) developed urticaria at 16 months and was hospitalized at 22 months. Another client in the same study was hospitalized for six weeks after developing a lung infection and when she was released from hospital she refused to talk to anyone. These researchers interpreted the mutistic response of the girl as a reaction to the separation from her mother, and as an attempt by the child to punish her parents for hospitalizing her.

In reviewing the medical history of one of their clients, Kaplan and Escoll (1973) reported that a young child they treated for elective mutism developed colic and vomiting before the onset of elective mutism. At age eight the child had unsubstantiated rheumatic fever and at age 15, the same client was admitted to a psychiatric unit because of hysterical ataxia following an appendectomy. The mother of another child in the same study, died suddenly when the daughter was twelve. The girl attempted suicide several times; the first attempt occurred at age nine.

Acute bronchitis was noted in a 10-day-old infant who later developed elective mutism (Morris, 1953). The same child also experienced extremely rough treatment by a neighbour who took the child to kindergarten. The clinician suggested that the social fears exhibited by the child originated with this event. In another case study Morris noted that his client was exposed to air raids at age three and became enuretic at age eight. Radford (1977) reported that the brain damage at birth of one child he treated for elective mutism may have been exacerbated by head-banging when the child was two years old. The female elective mute studied by Chethik (1973) developed several unhealthy reactions at 16 months of age including a severe feeding problem, hostility toward a new baby, and increased dependency on the mother.

INTERPLAY OF GEOGRAPHY AND LANGUAGE OF ORIGIN

Place of residence may have a bearing on elective mutism. For example, Morin *et al.* (1982) treated an electively mute male from a remote rural area and found that his family had few social contacts due to their physical isolation. Similarly, Morris (1953) noted that the family he dealt with preferred solitude and did not mix with neighbours. The family was also noted for frequent changes in places of residence. Nolan and Pence (1970) claimed that the family had moved frequently during the first two years of the electively mute child's life. Radford (1977) indicated that insularity was a characteristic of the family of the elective mute he treated. The closed nature of the family involving the restriction of social contacts to relatives and close friends was observed by Wassing (1970) in his investigation. The couple in the Halpern *et al.* (1971) study were described as being isolated, not only in their social relations with neighbours but they even remained aloof from their children. The parents of the clients treated by Friedman and Karagan (1973) were described as being socially withdrawn and shy.

Bradley and Sloman (1975) used the notion of "culture shock" to explain the acquisition of elective mutism among children of immigrants who did not speak the language of the region. Such children may be simultaneously exposed to a new place of residence as well as the task of learning a new language. The adjustment of the children and whether or not they will attempt to learn and speak the new language depends on the expectations the parents communicate to their children.

DISPARITY OF PHYSIQUE

Morris (1953) observed that the unusual physical appearance of the child he treated was correlated with being teased and bullied by other children. His discussion of what he termed "disparity of physique" did not, however, relate as much to the physical appearance of the child as to the behavior of family members which was judged by the community to be "different" or unusual.

Kupietz and Schwartz (1982) reported that the four-year-old boy they treated had a prominent upper lip, and a lower molar and upper canine that were abnormal in gross morphologic features. The boy walked with a limp; the right leg was slightly shorter than the left and the right foot was smaller than the left foot.

The unusual appearance of a child (including perhaps the wearing of clothing very different from the other children) makes a child highly visible to the other children. A child's highly visible appearance together with the fact that a child comes from a rural setting in which family histories are known by the majority of the other children contributes to making the child a target of abuse.

MOUTH TRAUMA

Wright (1968) and an earlier work by Parker *et al.* (1960) reported that histories of electively mute children frequently indicated "mouth injury" or "mouth trauma" coinciding with the time of learning to speak. Other clinicians (Pustrom and Speers, 1964) also found evidence for a mouth trauma – elective mutism connection and described the form of the mouth trauma as follows:

The mother was often intolerant of Bobby's incessant chatter, and frequently told him to "shut up" or slapped him on the mouth (p. 289).

Parker *et al.* (1960) claim that the onset of elective mutism may coincide with a trauma which occurs during the critical time that the child is learning to speak. These researchers found that the trauma often takes the form of an assault to the mouth (e.g., "shut up" and slapping the child across the mouth). More important, however, for the development of elective mutism is the reduction in the reciprocal mother-child verbal communications. These reciprocal exchanges draw the child's attention to communication, and the near-absence of communication may favor the development of elective mutism.

DISCUSSION

In the patient described by Pustrom and Speers (1964) the child's talking met with negatively reinforcing consequences. Nonetheless, as Browne *et al.* (1963) observed, electively mute individuals "can and do speak to certain specific people, usually one or both parents, and sometimes peers" (p. 605). Their statement corresponds to the observations in the majority of the published reports as well as the guidelines in *DSM–3–R* and *DSM–IV Options*. But in children who had been slapped across the mouth for excessive chatter, it would be expected that they would elect to use silence at home and to talk outside the home. Perhaps silence is used selectively at home, to stop annoying the parents and to avoid talking about topics which make the parents uncomfortable.

PERSONS TO WHOM ELECTIVELY MUTE PERSONS SPEAK

I have attempted to summarize the information about the settings and people to whom electively mute persons speak. A review of published studies yielded the following major trends:

- Electively mute persons usually speak within the home to immediate family members (Barlow *et al.*, 1986; Bozigar and Hansen, 1984; Brown and Doll, 1988; Carr and Afnan, 1989; Coutts, 1985; Furst, 1989; Kehle *et al.*, 1990; Kupietz and Schwartz, 1982; Lachenmeyer and Gibbs, 1985; Pigotte and Gonzales, 1987). The pre-1980 literature also shows that speaking to family members in the home is typical of silence users.
- There are a few studies (e.g., (Albert-Stewart, 1986; Atoynatan, 1986; Kaplan and Escoll, 1973) in which silence users were reported to be selectively mute to one parent – without exception the target of the silence was the father.
- Several studies mention the conditions under which silence users will speak in the family home. One of the major factors which will invoke the silence user role is the presence of strangers and non-family members (e.g., Crumley, 1990; Elson *et al.*, 1965; Landgarten, 1975; Morin *et al.*, 1982).
- Although electively mute individuals are usually verbal at home, there are a small number of studies which indicate that electively mute children do talk to selected individuals outside the family home. Browne *et al.* (1963) mentioned that their patient talked to neighbourhood children in the absence of adults. Colligan *et al.* (1977) observed that their clients spoke to younger children and to one friendly male neighbour. Nolan and Pence (1970) claimed that their patient spoke to a female neighbour and her children. Furthermore, Tanash (1986) indicated that one of their clients spoke to an "older boy" while a second spoke to children at school. An early study by Reed (1963) reported that his electively mute adolescent spoke to one teacher and one peer.

Discussion

These unique cases – electively mute children who *do talk* to selected individuals outside the home – are the most intriguing of the results of my review. Significant questions are prompted by these observations. What is it about the characteristics of these individuals which leads them to participate in conversations with people who are not members of the immediate family? Would it not be advantageous to identify the verbal and nonverbal behaviors which characterize these encounters? What does the onset of these speaking episodes with outsiders look like? Who initiates and stops the dialogue? What do the participants do or talk about? What is the nature of the psychological relationship between the silence user and the other person? Would the relationship be characterized as democratic or authoritarian? Or would observations reveal that the encounters with the outsider approximated a friendship relationship? *Direct observation* of the behavior of the participants would readily yield answers to these questions. The participants could also be *interviewed* to determine *why* the silence users talked to them and not to other people. To my knowledge, applied researchers have not addressed this type of "unique case" yet valuable information would undoubtedly result from this approach.

TELEPHONE USE

Although it has been reported that electively mute children do not speak on the telephone, several studies have indicated that electively mute children readily use the telephone (Ambrosino and Allessi, 1979). Browne *et al.* (1963) observed that their male electively mute client would talk on the telephone to individuals that he would refuse to talk to in person. In another study (Norman and Broman, 1970), the child routinely answered the telephone at home. Morris (1953) described how an elementary school child talked to her mother on the telephone in the principal's office. This was significant because this was one of the first occasions that the child was observed to speak in the presence of a non-family member.

There are several studies in which the telephone played a role in treatment. In Chethik's (1973) study, a young electively mute female expressed an interest in using the telephone during treatment and calls were first made to relatives. The mother's reaction, however, was to curtail the number and length of calls because she felt that the child was disturbing the relatives. Sluckin (1977) used the telephone with one of the two children she treated but it was limited to talking with the child several times over a two week period at the beginning of treatment. Except for the Rosenberg and Lindblad (1978) study, the telephone seems to have been used more by accident than being purposively included as a part of treatment. They used a telephone in combination with puppets in treating a little boy. The therapist called and the child readily talked to the therapist through the medium of the puppet.

SOUND OF ELECTIVE MUTE'S OWN VOICE

It is important to determine the child's appraisal of the sound of his own voice before proceeding with treatment. The reason for this is to avoid emphasizing, in the early stages of treatment, activities which might be experienced negatively by the client. For example, it would be inadvisable to play back a tape of a child's conversation if the child is fearful of or dislikes the sound of his voice. This position is supported by Browne *et al.* (1963):

The electively mute child seems to be afraid of the sound of his own voice. One of our patients had to give a talk at school. She taped the material, took the recorder to school, and fled from the room after turning on the tape recorder (p. 608).

In the above example, the electively mute child would have been less fearful if the tape had been played initially in the presence of the therapist and trusted classmates or teachers. Bednar (1974) presents a contrasting view. He reported that the child he worked with enjoyed listening to recordings of his own voice. In fact, Bednar reported that giving the child an opportunity to listen to his own voice constituted an effective reinforcer for speaking.

CHAPTER 5

PSYCHOSOCIAL CHARACTERISTICS OF
ELECTIVELY MUTE PERSONS
PART 2

IDENTICAL TWINS

Two female identical twins did not speak in class from primary to second semester of the sixth grade (Mora *et al.*, 1962). The mother was not seriously concerned about the girl's problem and applied for treatment only at the school's insistence. The mutism was first observed when they were being cared for by their paternal grandmother during an illness of their maternal grandmother. The mother attributed her daughters silence to shyness. The mother claimed that she did not feel like talking about unpleasant topics but she "didn't have the courage of the girls not to talk" (Mora *et al.*, 1962).

Intellectual Assessment

Despite the fact that the clients did not respond verbally, there is virtually no discussion of the difficulties that the examiners experienced in assessing these individuals. One notable exception is the early study by Mora *et al.* (1962) in which they indicated that although their clients were mute during testing, they cooperated by writing their responses to the questions in the verbal subtests of the WISC. With few exceptions, the majority of the studies indicate that the silence users were of average intelligence. The potential for above average academic performance based on formal intellectual assessments and/or school-based achievement was mentioned by Wassing (1973), Nolan and Pence (1970), Marcus *et al.* (1973), Landgarten (1975), Van der Kooy and Webster (1975), Colligan *et al.* (1977), Lipton (1980), Croghan and Craven (1982), Lachenmeyer and Gibbs (1985), and Beck and Hubbard (1987). In spite of the recognized observation that electively mute children ordinarily speak at home to one or both parents, there is only one study (Wulbert *et al.*, 1973) which used the parents to *administer* a formal assessment of intelligence. Furthermore, this study highlights the fact that educators, counsellors and health professionals have generally neglected to involve the people to whom the silence user talks in obtaining information about his or her target behavior problem.

I am puzzled why intelligence data was obtained for clients suspected of being electively mute in that there seems to be little if any connection between the intellectual status, the treatment expectations and the treatment regimen itself. Information about the child's achievement in school, however, could have important implications for the child's electing to be a silence user. This information, however, could ordinarily be obtained from the child's teachers without formal testing. Since, by definition, the majority of electively mute persons speak to certain people in at least one setting, it would be more relevant to monitor the individual's speech and language in the setting in which he elects to speak. Information on frequency, duration of episodes of spontaneous speech, and the proportion of spontaneous and prompted speech would seem to yield more useful data for setting realistic treatment expectations and designing treatments than intelligence data.

One could argue, however, that information about the client's intelligence is important in the assessment phase of the intervention because a low level of intellectual functioning in addition to the silence user role makes it difficult for the therapist (or mediator) to interview the person. Information about a person's intellectual functioning (or the more readily obtainable data on school achievement) is therefore useful for individualizing the format of the interview. The techniques of interviewing persons who are intellectually impaired may be useful for questioning silence users. The responses of less-educated adults and intellectually impaired persons are likely to vary depending on how questions are structured (e.g., open-ended vs. "closed" or checklist questions) and the options for recording the answers.

Open-ended questions are less effective than other types of questioning techniques. One can, of course, make it easier for intellectually impaired persons to respond by using examples in open-ended questions. For example, the open-ended question, "Do you talk to anyone at school? If yes, Who do you speak to?" might be replaced with "Do you talk to anyone at school, such as your teacher or the person who sits in front of you? If yes, which ones?" Other more useful alternatives of questioning intellectually impaired persons include verbal and pictorial multiple choice questions (Sigelman et al., 1982).

SALIENT CHARACTERISTICS OF THE MOTHER

Use of Silence

The mothers of electively mute children tend to use silence as a way of coping with their children's misbehavior and their husband's unreasonable demands. For example, Ambrosino and Alessi (1979) drew attention to one mother who used silence for coping with a child who was habitually truant. In an attempt to prevent relationships from further deteriorating in the family, the mother refused to discuss problems affecting the family. The mother believed that if she was silent, the situation would not worsen and she would be safe. One woman in the Kaplan and Escoll (1973) study expressed her anger toward her husband by refusing to speak to him for weeks at a time.

Dependency

Browne *et al.* (1963) reported that a mother of an electively mute child in their study had difficulty expressing her feelings. The only emotion she could clearly identify was anger. In addition, she developed a symbiotic-like relationship with her son in response to her disappointment with her husband. In another study Rosenberg and Lindblad (1978) reported that the mother aligned herself with her electively mute son to retaliate against her husband because of his minimal involvement with the children.

Passivity

Crema and Kerr (1978) indicated that the mother of their electively mute client very reluctantly confronted her husband. A study by Elson *et al.* (1965) confirms the tendency of wives to inhibit expressing anger to the husband. They claimed that the women's inhibition of anger was related to fear of abandonment.

Resentment

Meijer (1979) described two mothers who felt very resentful toward their husbands because of their constant need for admiration and because the mothers received very little concern from them in return. Another mother in the same study was resentful of her husband because she invested more time and energy in pleasing her husband than he did in pleasing her. Similarly, Mora *et al.* (1962) described the woman's attitude toward her husband as "hopeless and resentful." Salfield (1950) hinted at the resentful attitude of the mother in their study when they claimed that she tended "to [silently] harbour a grudge against society."

Behavior Management of Children

In a study by Pustrom and Speers (1964), a mother was reported to be intolerant of the child's incessant chatter. She discouraged the child from talking by slapping him on the mouth and telling him to shut-up. An art therapist (Landgarten, 1975) observed that the mother of the child she treated was very critical and demanding of the child's behavior. The mother prematurely terminated treatment and eventually abandoned the family.

Dominance in the Mother

Morris (1953) described a mother who was both dominant and aggressive when dealing with family members. The mother is also mentioned as being the dominant person in the family in the Zondlo and Scanlan (1983) study. Furst (1989) is the only researcher to use other than clinical impressions to support the notion of the dominance of the mother. This method is based on a sign approach to clinical assessment in which performance on a paper and pencil test is suggestive of the picture of interactions in the family. The sign approach is in contrast to the behavior sample approach which is based on direct observation.

The graphic representation of the 11-year-old patient depicted her mother as a large circle at the top of a retaining circle with her father depicted below by a much smaller circle. Beneath the father, in chronological order were circles of equal size, representing her brothers. At the bottom of the retaining circle she placed her only sister in an even smaller circle, and finally in the smallest circle of all, she placed herself. All circles were equidistant to one other except the one representing the child's mother, which was notably apart from, and above, all the rest. According to Furst (1989), this was a "sign" of a maternal-parental family dominance and his hypothesis was supported by direct observation.

Family Secrets

Pustrom and Speers (1964) described a mother who repeatedly cautioned her child not to talk to his paternal grandmother because she feared that the grandmother might reveal family secrets to the psychiatrist the grandmother was seeing. In the same article, the authors described another mother who dominated conversations to avoid being asked questions. These researchers found that a fear of revealing family secrets was common to mothers of their three young electively mute clients. They claimed that:

A factor common to all three mothers concerned conflicts about talking, primarily over revealing "family secrets." Gwen's mother repeatedly expressed her concern that the children and her husband "might say the wrong thing," so that hostile thoughts and feelings toward a superior, as well as sexual knowledge, might be revealed. Bobby's mother expressed concern that he might divulge his knowledge of the quarrels between herself and her husband. Johnny's mother expressed concern that he might indiscriminately reveal his knowledge of his parent's sexual life, as well as the illegitimacy scandal, should he learn of it. His continuous chatter when he was around her suggested to her that he might chatter elsewhere and this represented a constant threat to her.

We speculate that when the child entered nursery school, kindergarten, or grade school, the anger engendered in the child by the disruption of the mutual, infantile dependency relationship with mother resulted in the sadistic wish to "tell on mother" and thus attack her. However, such a sadistic impulse threatened the child with the possibility of total abandonment, and the child compromised by elective mutism (p. 293).

Implications for the Development of Elective Mutism

The mother has a need to escape from a disappointing marital relationship by fostering an unusual dependence on her child. The child in turn begins to control the mother and to make excessive demands on her. In some instances, electively mute children become almost totally controlling and oppositional. This carries over into their interactions outside the home. While some of these children appear to be fearful of entering new relationships, Subak *et al.* (1982) claim that the controlling element appears to be dominant.

SALIENT CHARACTERISTICS OF THE FATHER

The following publications are a representative sample of the characteristics of fathers of electively mute children:
- Tests the limits of therapy (such as being late for appointments, and non-payment of bills for treatment) (Browne *et al.*, 1963).
- Avoids discussing the child's elective mutism and refuses to believe that there could be a psychological reason for the mutism (Elson *et al.*, 1965).
- Shows intolerance of the child's refusal to talk at school (Rosenberg *et al.*, 1978).
- Reinforces wife's overprotectiveness with child (Wassing, 1973).
- Critical of children and spouse (Meijer, 1979).
- Punishes wife by refusing to talk to her for long period of time (Browne *et al.*, 1963).
- Emotionally distant, insensitive, unavailable and unaware of family and child's mutism (Ruzicka and Sackin, 1974).
- Quiet and silent at home (Morris, 1953).
- Overly work-oriented and not available to his family (Chethik, 1973).
- Avoids conflicts and expression of emotion (Wassing, 1973).
- Quiet with stammer/stutter (Sluckin, 1977; Meijer, 1979).
- Quiet individual (Colligan *et al.*, 1977).
- Perceives being dominated by wife (Kaplan and Escoll, 1973).
- Passive (Pustrom and Speers, 1964).
- Spokesman and protector of family (Halpern *et al.*, 1971).

- Public speaker enthusiastically engaged in outside activities (Meijer, 1979).
- Talkative and manipulative of people (Meijer, 1979).
- Intense fear of speaking in public (Pustrom and Speers, 1964).
- Exhibits depression and suicidal behavior. Morris (1953), for example, reported that the fathers of two out of the six children he treated had committed suicide.
- Tense and anxious (Reed, 1963).

The father may be less talkative and involved in the affairs of the family but this should not be confused with lack of personal power or ineffectiveness in exercising control (Bly, 1990). Bly makes this insightful statement in response to the stereotype of masculine passivity in the family:

Each father inherits thousands of years of cunning and elaborate fatherhood. *An apparently weak father can control the entire family from beneath with his silences.* Should the father be an alcoholic, his alcoholism may be a massive operation, carried out with Napoleonic thoroughness, so that he rules his house by the most economical means. The Destructive Father does not give energy to those in his family but draws it out of them into some black hole he shelters in himself. He draws it out steadily, as the great tyrants we know of draw it from their citizens (Bly, 1990, p. 115).

In summarizing, it appears that no clear personality pattern may be drawn for the fathers of elective mutes. Generally speaking, however, they seem to assume a passive role in family affairs. In spite of the intuitive appeal of Bly's proposition, the use of silence as a punishment or manipulative device is rarely noted about the father in the published accounts of elective mutism.

CHAPTER 6

PSYCHOSOCIAL CHARACTERISTICS OF
ELECTIVELY MUTE PERSONS
PART 3

DEPENDENCY

A number of writers have commented on the dependency of electively mute children. Bauermeister and Jemail (1975) found a pronounced dependency on the mother by her electively mute child. The child in the case study by Wassing (1973) demonstrated extreme dependency on his mother, even for toilet training. Sluckin (1977) described a female child that she treated for elective mutism as being very "clingy" to her mother.

RELATION TO BEHAVIORAL INHIBITION

Behavioral inhibition is a synonym for what is commonly referred to as shyness. Morris (1953) and Reed (1963) observed shyness in three out of four of their case studies. A report by Meijer (1979) indicated shyness in four out of five of his patients. It is widely mentioned in the elective mutism literature that there is minimal or no eye contact in communication (Elson et al., 1965; Friedman and Karagan, 1973; Marcus et al., 1973; Bednar, 1974; Colligan et al., 1977; Sluckin, 1977; Crema and Kerr, 1978; Rosenberg and Lindblad, 1978).

Electively mute children are frequently depicted as being shy by therapists, teachers and parents. The characteristics of shyness are not discussed in the elective mutism literature but it appears that the shyness involves social fears including fears of rejection. If fear is considered a significant component of shyness, an operational definition of shyness as a characteristic of elective mutism would have to delineate three components of fear. First, information would have to be obtained about whether or not the individual verbalized his fear of speaking. A statement such as "I am afraid of speaking" illustrates this component. A second feature usually referred to as the motoric component of fear should be assessed. An example of this would be the child's retreating to his room or becoming silent whenever a stranger entered the room. Finally, a comprehensive assessment of fear should include information about various physiological responses such as stomach upset, excessive perspiration, difficulty in breathing and increased heart rate that the client reports experiencing before or during speaking episodes.

Kagan et al. (1987) researched predictors of inhibited and uninhibited children. They found that very young infants do not usually avoid un-familiar people or objects but observed that infants assessed at 9 or 14 months arched their backs away from unfamiliar people or objects. These researchers defined fear in young children as crying when encountering an unfamiliar object, e.g., a black box with a hole in it, an event, a person, or the young children's failure to approach an unfamiliar person following an invitation to do so such as offering the child a toy. The following observation of an electively mute child (Reid *et al.*, 1973) coincides with behavioral inhibition – "Sally, aged six, would speak to no one but her immediate family, not even to a family member when a stranger was present" (p. 152). Kagan *et al.* concluded that behavioral inhibition may be a product of specific experiences, independent of any temperamental bias. They also claimed that a small number of these children have a predisposition to be behaviorally inhibited given specific environmental conditions. In observing children at 4 months, 9 months and 14 months, they observed that high motoric activity and frequent crying were correlated with behavioral inhibition during childhood.

According to Kagan *et al.*, *one of the most sensitive indices of inhibition was the reluctance to talk to an unfamiliar person.* The researchers used latency of response as a measure of reluctance to talk. They found that the majority of the uninhibited five-year-olds emitted the second spontaneous verbal response within three minutes of meeting the unfamiliar person and emitted 40 or more comments within a 90-minute observation period. In contrast, the inhibited children of the same age did not emit a spontaneous comment until approximately ten minutes had elapsed and, on average, they spoke less than 10 times. Kagan and Snidman (1991) claimed that the mothers of the less inhibited children, compared with those who had remained inhibited, had helped their children to overcome their inhibition by introducing peers into the home and teaching them coping skills for social fears. Kagan and Snidman (1991) also found that inhibited children exhibited a higher and more stable heart rate than less inhibited children when faced with an unfamiliar person, object or event. They argued that "the threshold of responsivity in limbic and hypothalamic structures to unfamiliarity and challenge is tonically lower for inhibited than for uninhibited children" (p. 1459).

STUBBORNNESS

Stubbornness seems to be a feature of elective mutism. Stubbornness is often described in various studies as an unwillingness to yield and may manifest itself as passive resistance (Nolan and Pence, 1970). Chethik (1973) mentioned passivity that boarders on obstinacy, while Crema and Kerr (1978) described a female electively mute individual and her father as demonstrating "extreme stubbornness." The tendency of an electively mute person to become "difficult" when he did not get his own way was observed by Radford (1977). Pustrom and Speers (1964) and Rosenbaum and Kellman (1973) briefly referred to the stubbornness of their clients.

AGGRESSION

Browne *et al.* (1963) equated the electively mute child's banging on steel cabinets and windows with his fists in therapy as behavioral indicators of "angry feelings." Nolan and Pence (1970) mentioned a female elective mute's aggressiveness with peers. In addition, their observations of electively mute female twins determined that the "symptom [mutism] is not only a way of passively expressing hostility, but a means of controlling people, of keeping them at a distance and resisting outside influence" (Mora *et al.*, 1962). One of two types of elective mutism described by Reed (1963) deals with attention-getting, manipulative children with aggressive tendencies. Zondlo and Scanlan (1983) spoke of frequent temper tantrums in their treatment of a deaf electively mute adult female. Halpern *et al.* (1971) also commented on temper tantrums and on the difficulty the parents experienced in handling these episodes.

PROTECTION FROM OTHER PROBLEMS

Weininger (1987) indicates that his two patients (aged six and seven) exhibited reading difficulties. The two children developed many somatic complaints of a nonorganic origin *after* they started to talk. In another case, a 10-year-old boy became very depressed and withdrawn, failing all his school work after he started to talk outside the home.

FAMILY PROBLEMS

Kaplan and Escoll (1973) noted that the marital relationship in one of the two families they discussed was characterized by disappointment and hostility. The relationship between the daughter and father, however, was extremely positive; in fact so much so that the researchers described greetings between the two as similar to "reuniting lovers." The 12-year-old girl in the Kaplan and Escoll (1973) study rarely spoke to her father because "both had agreed that there was nothing to say." The estrangement between the two was visible before her mother's death but increased after her death. Sexual disharmony, financial difficulties and arguments over the husband's alcoholism were discussed by Pustrom and Speers (1964).

In another case, they related a conflict between the parents over procreation. Crema and Kerr (1978) reported that the father of their client regularly "burst into rage at a moment's notice." Generally, the mother responded with "silence" while the electively mute child exhibited no fear of her father's outbursts and frequently told him to "shut-up." Morris (1953) claimed that family problems might lead to elective mutism, especially in a rural community. He suggested that the use of silence lessened the attention the client received and this probably reduced the real or anticipated rejection by community members.

SEXUAL ABUSE AND ELECTIVE MUTISM

Susan Forward and Craig Buck (1988) in the *Betrayal of Innocence: Incest and Its Significance* speak of the spectrum of the "silent partner" in which involvement of the nonabusive caretaker can range from ignoring signs of incest to subtly promoting it. Forward and Buck claim that the mother communicates to her children by her nonverbal behavior and sometimes in words that she is unable to protect them. In such families, the children are frequently observed to protect the mother by withholding any information which would upset the mother or the family. By abdicating her personal power, the mother becomes unable to protect her children.

Reed (1963) provides one of the few accounts which reported an elective mutism – sexual abuse connection. This was a case of sexual abuse by a peer. A 13-year-old girl was referred to the clinic by the mother who felt that the child was becoming progressively unhappy. She also claimed that the child had been happy until the age of nine, when she had been sexually assaulted by a 16-year-old boy. Several months later, however, the mother admitted that the story had been based on a retrospective interpretation of what might well have been an innocuous event in order to explain her child's behavior.

ELECTIVE MUTISM: AN INTEGRATIVE RESPONSE

Kaplan and Escoll (1973) asserted that silence resolved the problem of relating to the opposite-sexed parent while simultaneously adhering to the family regulation against forming significant relationships with anyone outside the family.

Silence solved the problem of separation, the problem of the prohibition against the expression of anger, and the problem of excess stimulation of sexual feelings toward the parent of the opposite sex. The adolescent could remain in the family, but deny her entrapment by not talking. She could leave the family, but deny her separation from them by not talking with her peers. She could both deny to herself and to other members of the family any feelings of anger toward them. At the same time she could provoke them into angry tirades toward her because of her silence. Anger on the father's part would make the threat of sexuality easier to tolerate because it made for greater psychological distance between them.

Similarly, the patient's silence partially solved these same problems for the family. As long as the patient was silent, the family rules against separation, and against the expression of anger and sexuality, could be maintained to some degree. Furthermore, the patient provided the family with a scapegoat. When the patient began to speak, however, the threat of breaking one or more of these rules became imminent. The parents' paradoxical increase in anger and disorganization as the patient began to improve may be understood in terms of this threat (pp. 67–68).

Kaplan and Escoll emphasized that a "closed-family" situation discouraged the development of heterosexual interests outside the family and this, together with the prohibition of expressing anger, made it difficult for the girls to defend themselves against sexual advances by the father.

DISCUSSION

The research indicates that the mothers show a combination of dependency and lack of assertiveness in the family and they attempt to allay themselves with one or more of the children. This picture is complicated by the observation that many electively mute children are themselves shy and dependent. They often become dependent on the mother and yet she is ill-equipped to give the support desired by the child because of her problematic relationship with her husband. The fathers of these children are frequently pictured as being minimally involved with the children. They often exhibit what might be described as a strong-silent stance which is intimidating to both the mother and children. The communication pattern of both parents in refusing to talk about events which are troubling the family is perhaps adopted by the child who exhibits elective mutism either as an expression of family turmoil or as a coping response to reduce anxiety.

The children or adolescents are not in a position to withdraw physically from the home because they need the protection and support, albeit minimal in some instances, that they are receiving from the family. The withdrawal, therefore, is exhibited in withdrawal of verbal communication rather than physical withdrawal. The review of the psychosocial literature shows that there are several models for non-physical withdrawal in the client's family: (1) staying with the family while not asking for anything, (2) staying with the family while not talking about events which are troubling the family – "keeping the peace" by becoming a silence user, (3) staying with the family and remaining silent about contentious issues to reduce fears of abandonment by one or both parents and (4) staying with the family and attempting to avoid real or anticipated negative consequences by maintaining family secrets through being silent. The father also models a strong silent stance which conveys that it is possible to be a member of the family without becoming involved in the affairs of the family.

Children cannot help but be influenced by these social learning experiences. Although the electively mute children may fear events in school, they nonetheless attend school rather than physically absent themselves from school. The children, therefore, conform to the requirement of attending school but avoid involving themselves in speaking-related activities. This pattern is very similar to what the children observe at home and may help to explain why the children do not withdraw physically from school. The fact that the electively mute individual speaks in one situation and not in another setting could also be partly explained by the relative probability of punishments and rewards in the two settings. In one setting the client can "get away with" electing to be silent while in another setting he would be punished for the silence. Teachers may even believe that the children's silence is typical of their communication style in other settings. It is also possible that in one setting the probability of receiving reinforcement for being silent is greater than in other settings.

REACTIONS TO ELECTIVE MUTISM

Silence User's Response to Therapist's Verbalizations

Shreeve (1991) said that when his four-year-old female client began to talk, she responded to his verbalizations by covering her ears, laughing, and continuing to talk as if she had not heard the therapist. Shreeve argued that the behavior change involved a substitution of not listening for not talking.

Reactions of School Personnel

Browne *et al.* (1963) observed that the reactions of teachers follow a predictable sequence. I have called the three phases discussed by Browne *et al.* identification, frustration-anger, and ultimatum. During the *identification phase* teachers often make no attempt to indicate to the children that they are expected to talk. Teachers of electively mute children frequently accept them as non-speaking individuals. According to Browne *et al.*, the length of the identification phase varies from a few months to several years.

During the *frustration-anger phase*, overt attempts are made to encourage the child to talk. The child usually responds to these attempts with resistance and panic and an impasse is reached between the family and the school. Because electively mute children talk at home the parents cannot understand why they do not talk at school (Browne *et al.*, 1963). An unco-operative relationship between the school and the home mitigates against the effective treatment of elective mutism. Rosenbaum and Kellman (1973) described a scenario in which the school personnel felt the mother was inaccessible, and the parents claimed that the teachers were not sufficiently concerned about the daughter's problem of elective mutism. During the *ultimatum-phase* teachers insist that the child either talk or risk not being promoted to the next grade (Browne *et al.*, 1963) and presumably punish-ment of various sorts might also be threatened or administered.

Bednar (1974) described the unfavourable reaction of a teacher who was asked to become involved in the treatment of an electively mute child. According to the author, he was reluctant to work with the client because of his low tolerance level and because the task itself was time consuming. Ambrosino and Alessi (1979) reported that one child's kindergarten teacher denied that her student was a silence user. The teacher noticed the lack of speech but considered it a minor problem. Another teacher, however, claimed that her student's elective mutism was caused by "some deep psychological problems, since she was so terribly frightened of the world that she was unwilling to answer even the most simple questions" (p. 387). A study by Mora *et al.* (1962) however, describes a contrasting approach. In this study, school authorities clearly indicated to the mute twins and their parents that they were expected to talk or be withdrawn from school. This power ploy immediately elicited the cooperation of the twins.

Norman and Broman (1970) reported that speech therapists, school psychologists and other professionals had unsuccessfully attempted to treat an electively mute male child but were very pessimistic concerning the likelihood of success regardless of the treatment used. The teachers, however, who received training in the principles of behavior therapy assumed responsibility for the boy's treatment in the school setting and were successful. Wassing (1973) emphasized that it is important to extend treatment beyond the mental health clinic and to obtain the assistance of the teachers in implementing treatment. Several authors affirmed the value of teacher co-operation during therapy carried out in a school setting (Crema and Kerr, 1978; Dmitriev and Hawkins, 1973; Halpern *et al.*, 1971; Lipton, 1980; Marcus *et al.*, 1973; Morin *et al.*, 1982; Nolan and Pence, 1970). In each of these studies, the teacher acted wholly or in part as a behavior change agent. Salfield (1950) reported that untrained school personnel unsuccessfully attempted to elicit speech. In another study, Van der Kooy and Webster (1975) reported that the teacher tried unsuccessfully to force an electively mute child to speak. The specific methods used were not mentioned in the Salfield (1950) and Van der Kooy and Webster (1975) studies.

Discussion

An electively mute child frequently attends school for several years without talking. This implies that the teachers have been patient and may even have individualized their teaching methods and learning materials so that the child could progress without speaking. This approach, although extremely caring, does not get the child to speak and perhaps it is detrimental because it does not encourage verbal interpersonal communication.

Reactions of Peers

From the point of view of both assessment and treatment, it may be advantageous to address the following three questions: (1) Are electively mute children generally accepted by their peers? Is the child invited to join group activities by the other children? (2) Do peers reinforce the child's elective mutism? If so, what is the nature of the reinforcement? and (3) Are the peers functioning in a way which might be described as therapeutic? For example, when the child does speak, do they listen? Do they reinforce the child for speaking? If so, what are the nature of the rewards?

Studies frequently report that the reactions of peers positively reinforce the elective mutism. Wassing (1973) said that the tolerance shown by peers often made it unnecessary for electively mute children to talk. Colligan *et al.* (1977) reported that classmates frequently explained to strangers that their friend does not talk. Lipton (1980), Rosenbaum and Kellman (1973) reported that the classmates spoke on behalf of the electively mute child. Nolan and Pence (1970) indicated that the non-verbal communication of the female electively mute child they treated was reinforced by both teachers and students. Wassing (1973) asserted that his adolescent patient was accepted by the members of his peer group. This researcher said that:

John was well accepted by most of his group members. His persistent abstinence from speech was not seized upon by them as a motive for rejection or even teasing. Contrary to this he was generally respected, and his keeping silence was even met with [glowing] remarks (p. 78).

Wassing suggested that the peers were positively reinforcing the adolescent's silence user behavior. He claimed that:

The tolerance of his mates regarding his muteness, if not reinforcing the symptom, at least did not impose upon him the need for change. The respect that he received from his peers allowed him to continue his mutistic response pattern without having to fear that he would be rejected by the group because of this (p. 78).

The classmates of the six-year-old electively mute child described by Kehle *et al.* (1990) accepted him and even offered excuses for his non-verbal behavior and would often intercede on his behalf. Not all electively mute children are accepted by their peers. Ruzicka and Sackin (1974) state that elective mutes are sometimes teased and often ignored by their agemates. Sluckin (1977) similarly reports that children frequently do not want to associate or talk with electively mute peers. According to Wassing (1973), fellow pupils reacted negatively when they discovered that their friend could but did not speak. The use of silence in this case was viewed by the peers as arrogance and consequently the child was teased and ridiculed. In one study (Halpern *et al.*, 1971), it was suggested that if a child is teased because of a speech problem, such as stuttering, it may lead a child to avoid ridicule by becoming a silence user.

Physical and Nonverbal Presence in Elective Mutism

The study by Subak *et al.* (1982) addresses the issue of the verbal and physical presence of the person. The 15-year-old female treated by these clinicians exhibited school refusal (absenteeism) in addition to elective mutism. The adolescent client of Subak *et al.* (1982) responded to questions by nodding her head for "yes" or shrugging her shoulders for "don't know." These researchers, however, also identified occasions in which the person elected to be nonverbally silent.

Discussion

Subak *et al.* (1982) have raised an intriguing and important issue. They claimed that when provoked their adolescent client looked annoyed and temporarily stopped nonverbally communicating. Do electively mute patients stop nonverbally communicating as Subak *et al.* (1982) suggest? If this occurs, then it might be appropriate to use the term "visual silence" to describe "elective mutism equivalence" in nonverbal communication. Electing to be "visually silent," however, seems not to have been typical of their patient. But their observation does illustrate that elective mutism (electing to be verbally silent) and "visual silence" (electing to be "nonverbally silent") can be simultaneously present in the same person. This is a complicated issue, however, because ceasing to answer questions nonverbally could also be interpreted as disagreement or annoyance rather than the cessation of nonverbal communication. The observation of Subak *et al.* (1982) also raises the question as to whether it is possible to stop nonverbally communicating. The nonverbal communication may change but it is difficult to determine what the cessation of nonverbal communication would look like. An absence of nonverbal communication would only be a tenable proposition, however, if the nonverbal responses were seen as neutral because as soon as they are seen as having a positive or negative valence, we cannot argue for the absence of nonverbal communication.

While there may be intuitive appeal for the notion of nonverbal silence, the majority of electively mute children absent themselves verbally but not physically from the setting(s), in which they elect not to speak. Kehle *et al.* (1990) observed that the six-year-old boy they treated completely lacked any verbal interaction with his classmates or teachers. Yet, he appeared to enjoy the classroom experiences that did not require him to talk.

Electively mute persons are nonverbally absent yet physically present in the target settings. One might argue that electively mute children attend school because in the majority of jurisdictions school attendance is compulsory. Teachers are therefore required to monitor and record the attendance of each student. With the systematic monitoring of attendance, the physically absent student is readily identified.

While the majority of electively mute children comply with the compulsory attendance regulation, their excessive use of silence is not immediately apparent because of the very unobtrusive nature of the behavior problem. The "verbal absence" of children, therefore, goes unnoticed because their "silent presence" does not exceed the tolerance level of school personnel as much as the excessive verbal and motoric behavior of the other children which interferes with teaching and learning. Because of these reasons, expectations for the child to participate may be minimal especially if the achievement of the child in written work is satisfactory.

The silence user role does not seem to preclude involvement in a learning activity and hence the "verbally absent" child may go unnoticed or the child's use of silence may be inadvertently reinforced by teacher and peer attention. In addition, the anticipated or actual punishment for "verbal absence" is likely to be minimal or non-existent – and certainly one might speculate that the magnitude of threats or punishments would be substantially less than for behavior which disrupts teaching and the learning of other students.

CHAPTER 7

THEORIES OF ELECTIVE MUTISM

INTRODUCTION

The elective mutism literature focuses primarily on characteristics of specific patients and little has been done in systematic theory building. Theories about causes of elective mutism have not been confirmed by empirical research. Because of the scarcity of electively mute children, commonalities in the background of these children are difficult to investigate. Consequently, information must be abstracted from case studies (Brown and Doll, 1988). The purpose of this discussion is to develop a framework for diagnosing and treating elective mutism. Whenever possible, the theories are supported with the findings of researchers whose work suggests a learning theory framework.

FEAR-REDUCING ELECTIVE MUTISM AND ATTENTION-GETTING-MANIPULATIVE ELECTIVE MUTISM

Reed (1963) divided the cases of elective mutism into two distinct groups. One group was felt to have learned mutism as an attention-getting device and as an evasive form of behavior. These children were unlike the second group which used elective mutism as a fear-reducing mechanism. The attention-getting function indicates that the patient uses unadaptive silence to obtain positive reinforcement while the manipulative aspect signifies that the patient uses silence to exert control over others. Reports from family members indicate that the use of silence is followed by favorable outcomes for the patient. In addition to the primary gain of increased attention and controlling others, secondary gain is observable in the additional unsolicited special treats and activities which the silence user receives.

Research

A fear-reducing theory of elective mutism is supported by a number of scientist-practitioners. Krolian (1988) relates the anxiety-reduction function of the silence user role to treatment. Krolian claims that one of the major aims of treatment is to change the valence of speech from anxiety production to anxiety reduction. One of the four types of elective mutism delineated by Hayden (1980) is speech phobic mutism which is characterized by a fear of one's own voice. Pustrom and Speers (1964) discussed two of the fathers in their three case studies. One patient reported that his father spoke infrequently as a child. The patient also said that his father still had an intense fear of speaking in public. Ambrossino and Alessi (1979) indicated that the child which they treated stopped talking to reduce anxiety about her father's terminal illness. I believe that this patient's silence is a form of controlling negative or self-defeating sentences through thought-stopping. A thought-stopping formulation suggests that the fear-provoking stimulus is the message rather than the act of speaking. This intriguing issue has not been studied by elective mutism researchers.

Croghan and Craven (1982) concluded that elective mutism can be a form of speech-blocking. The patient may become anxious when speaking to persons other than family members and close friends and consequently elects not to speak.

Reed (1963) identified two types of elective mutism. Differences between the two types were based on the direct observation of clients' behavior during clinical interviews. According to Reed, if the silence has a fear-reducing function, the client will exhibit tense and watchful behaviors. The patient will be observed to be "selectively inactive" and the patient's nonverbal communication is readily interpreted as "avoidance" or "escape." The patient, for example, may exhibit gaze aversion. If the patient is a child, she will reluctantly enter the therapist's office and will resist separating herself from the adult who accompanies her. Such a patient will not exhibit exploratory behavior and will not play with toys or explore other things in view.

Evidence of fear-reducing elective mutism is also suggested in responses such as tics and jerky movements (Croghan and Craven, 1982). In addition, Wright (1968) elaborates on the interview behaviors of electively mute children. He found that young children had difficulty separating from their parents but older children separated easily although they appeared shy. The most noticeable response was that the children ignored the therapist and would not take part in nonverbal activities such as puzzles and games. When asked a question requiring a verbal response, they exhibited flushing and irregular breathing.

According to Reed (1963), if the function of the silence is attention-getting or to control others, the child will be observed to readily enter the therapist's office and separating from the guardian is not an observable issue. The patient does not confine herself to one spatial location but instead moves about in the therapy setting. The patient may be observed picking up various objects in the therapist's office. Other researchers also provide evidence for attention-getting-manipulative elective mutism. The electively mute children treated by Wilkins (1985) were described as "manipulative." Likewise, Hayden (1980) discusses symbiotic mutism which is characterized by a close relationship between the caretaker and the electively mute person and a submissive but manipulative relationship with others.

Similarly, Wright (1968) describes the relationship with the mother as dependent and ambivalent coupled with a need to be in control. Attention-getting and controlling electively mute adolescents may go to considerable ends before relinquishing control. In the Subak *et al.* (1982) study, it was necessary for the police to bring the client to the hospital. Weininger (1987) argues that by talking only to the mother, the child controls her. The child tells his or her mother what to do and, often, how to do things. The child is therefore able to maintain silence with others, and the manipulative behavior of the silence user role is reinforced by the response of the mother and others outside the family. Telephone use is rarely mentioned in the literature. Parker *et al.* (1960), however, reported that one of the children they treated would talk to anyone on the telephone. Unfortunately, it is not indicated if the child would initiate a telephone call or spontaneously answer the telephone. The researchers interpreted the child's attempts to get her therapist to telephone her as an attempt to control the therapist with whom the child refused to speak.

Krolian (1988) claimed that speaking has an anxiety-reducing function and an anxiety-producing function. Concerning the anxiety-reducing function, one can readily relate to talking to a friend when troubled and feeling less anxious after the conversation. She argued that one of the major aims of treatment is to change the "valence" of speaking from anxiety producing to anxiety reducing.

Discussion

I wish to add another dimension to Reed's discussion. Researchers have rarely discussed elective mutism from the perspective of the communication dyad which, in the case of elective mutism, consists of the silence user and the silence receiver. Potential reinforcers are readily hypothesized for silence users but it is difficult to identify the reinforcers for the silence receivers. Since there are few identifiable positive consequences for the silence receivers, the clinician must identify potentially reinforcing stimuli and assess the impact of the stimulus consequences through the medium of self-report. Silence receivers frequently give attention in the form of prompts to get silence users to talk. I also believe that the prompts topographically differ from one silence receiver to another. These prompts to elicit speech are similar, however, because they are correlated with internal statements of hope. Hope readily aligns with applied behavior analysis if it is equated with the expectation of a positive reinforcer (Stotland, 1969) which for the silence receiver is that the silence user will talk.

Based on the function served by the silence, Reed (1963) proposed a two-fold classification of elective mutism. In contrast to Reed, I believe that these two symptom functions might best be viewed on a continuum with the anxiety-reducing function identifying one end of the continuum and the manipulative-controlling function identifying the other end of the continuum. The rationale for this is that individuals may exhibit a combination of the two types. A more complex model acknowledging the above proposition is implied in the research of Lumb and Wolff (1988):

Although it may seem self-evident that children whose behavior is based on anxiety should be taught by methods such as successive approximation and those children whose behavior is based on manipulation should be taught by methods such as confrontation, matters are sometimes not quite so simple. It is quite possible for some children to be both anxious and manipulative and any teaching programme must therefore be sensitive and capable of rapid adjustment in the light of experience. On occasion a method such as successive approximation may be unsuccessful with a child whose withholding of speech is manipulative simply because it is a path that can be followed without losing face in front of a peer group. There are also occasions when it may be that an anxious child would best be helped by a teaching method based on confrontation (p. 22).

SELF-DESENSITIZATION THEORY

Pustrom and Speers (1964) suggest that the electively mute person speaks to people according to a subjective evaluation of danger that a situation represents. I shall attempt to develop this statement within a behavior therapy framework. A naturally occurring desensitization process may account for the recovery of those who do not receive formal treatment. Self-initiated desensitization, however, does not typically develop spontaneous speech. Instead, the individual's speech is characterized by reluctant communication – that is, the person will respond only if asked a question.

The process of naturally occurring desensitization does not have the precision of therapist designed desensitization and, therefore, the person's fear response may be extinguished to only a few speaking cues. There are three additional problems with self-initiated desensitization. First, the person may avoid speaking and this reinforces the silence user role if the avoidance behavior is associated with fear-reduction. Second, the individual may only momentarily speak but promptly escape by becoming silent. The *escape through silence* and the relief accompanying the escape response may reinforce the person's inappropriate use of silence because an escape response temporarily removes, terminates, or avoids personal discomfort. Third, the person's naturally occurring speaking models may exhibit fearless behaviors with which the speech phobic person cannot identify. Since fearless models do not provide visible coping characteristics, they do not help in extinguishing fears about speaking.

Nonetheless, if electively mute people use an effective desensitization strategy, manage to expose themselves to anxiety arousing speaking situations without escaping or avoiding them, and have good coping models for anxiety management, they may reduce the severity of their problem. Individuals who receive treatment for elective mutism have probably not adopted these adaptive responses.

TRAUMA THEORY

Parker *et al.* (1960) discussed the potential role of traumatic events in the development of elective mutism. They mentioned that elective mutism may be correlated with a history of mouth injury at the time the child was learning to speak. The child's chatter may be troublesome to people with a low threshold of annoyance and consequently they may instruct the child to "shut up" as well as give a slap across the mouth. I would like to briefly discuss the learning theory implications of the observations of Parker *et al.* This abusive approach may be adopted by parents who believe that a child should be "seen and not heard." The child, in such instances, learns to avoid or escape the aversive stimulation by becoming a silence user. While this role is helpful for the child, it does little to correct the emotionally and physically abusive behavior of the parents.

The above analysis would lead us to believe that elective mutism would occur in the home and that the child would speak outside the home. However, the reverse typically occurs. If speech-related trauma which occurs in the home has etiological importance for the development and/or maintenance of elective mutism, why does the electively mute response occur outside of the punishment context for speaking and why is it that the same electively mute person talks at home where speaking has been punished or negatively reinforced? The fact that the individual more often than not speaks inside the home in spite of traumatic speaking-related experiences initially seems to be difficult to account for by escape and avoidance learning. In the case of elective mutism, escape and avoidance learning would predict that the patient would not talk in the settings associated with the trauma.

Research

Halpern *et al.* (1971) suggested that early traumatic experiences were implicated in the etiology of elective mutism. Hayden (1980) referred to the role of traumatic events in his fourfold classification. In his system, traumatic mutism is a response to a traumatic event often accompanied by feelings of depression and social withdrawal. Depression in the families of electively mute patients has been reported in a number of studies. Rasbury

(1974) and Ruzicka and Sackin (1974) reported maternal depression in their case studies of electively mute children. In addition, Pustrom and Speers (1964) said that a father of one of their electively mute patients experienced periods of depression in which he withdrew and was socially uneasy. Kaplan and Escoll's (1973) case study of an electively mute youth and her widowed father indicated that the father was chronically depressed and both he and his daughter agreed "there was nothing to say." I believe that depression among family members should alert the clinician to the possibility that elective mutism may be a form of masked depression or a reaction to the depression of a family member.

Bullying at School

Physical, sexual and emotional abuse by peers is recognized as a problem in educational settings (Besag, 1989). Although the published literature about elective mutism does not refer to elective mutism as a response to abuse by peers, it could be an important factor contributing to the child's electing to be a silence user. This is an important consideration when it is observed that the child does not speak to other children during free time. By being silent the child may make himself less conspicuous and also lessen the likelihood of saying something which would result in being bullied. In such instances, electing to be silent could be viewed as a coping response to actual or anticipated bullying.

FAMILY MODELS OF COMMUNICATION

Goll (1979) offers a model of role-playing that occurs within the families of electively mute children. Goll argues that the families of electively mute children have minimal confidence in society and therefore insulate themselves from contacts with people outside the family.

Observational Learning Theory

Goll (1979) proposed a fourfold classification of roles in the families of elective mutes. First, there is the family member who is electively mute. Second, the electively mute patient may have had the opportunity to observe another family member who uses silence in inappropriate ways such as transitory stubbornness. Third, the role of a symbiotic partner is frequently observed in the families of elective mutes. According to Goll, the symbiotic partner is the individual, usually the mother, with whom the elective mute has an intense unhealthy attachment. I have observed in my clinical work that the silence user may speak to the mother but refuse to speak to the father. Research needs to focus on the role of symbiotic relationships in the development and maintenance of elective mutism. Fourth, the ghetto leader role refers to a family member who communicates distrust of the community and its official representatives to other family members. The implication seems to be that individuals who receive messages from influential family members that non-family members cannot be trusted may elect to become silence users.

I would like to briefly elaborate on Goll's discussion by suggesting several features of naturally occurring models which contribute to elective mutism. First, the patient may have been exposed to fearful models of escape or avoidance. Second, as has been mentioned in the discussion of the self-desensitization theory, the patient may have been exposed to fearless models rather than coping models. This means that the silence user received minimal information about managing speaking anxiety. Third, the patient may have experienced incomplete coping models. This means that the patient was exposed to models which communicated that speaking was desirable but they provided minimal information about social skills or guidelines for coping with fears about speaking. In addition, fearless models for talking may present the positive consequences of talking but they do not provide a conceptual map for dealing with inner fear responses. Many speaking models, unfortunately, provide guidelines for dealing with only one of the components of fear. In other words, the client is encouraged to display approach rather than avoidance or escape behavior. Although modeling of exposure to a fear stimulus provides therapeutically useful information, it does not necessarily provide observable guidelines for controlling internal statements of fear or unpleasant physiological manifestations of fear.

FAMILY SECRETS THEORY

Pustrom and Speers (1964) found that in the families of electively mute children the adult family members express exaggerated concern over revealing "family secrets" and of saying "the wrong thing." Since the majority of the families in Lesser-Katz's study (1988) depended on public assistance, it was important for them to keep other sources of income from becoming widely known. The presence in the home of the child's working father was often a secret. In many of these homes, violence inflicted by the man against the mother was common; this, too, was kept private.

Colligan *et al.* (1977) assert that family rules that discourage openness and exaggerate concerns about keeping secrets is correlated with elective mutism. This guideline against revealing family secrets is also mentioned by Wergeland (1979). This viewpoint is also reinforced by Meyer's (1984) observation of the families of elective mutes. He observed that suspiciousness of non-family members is coupled with fear of strangers and intense family loyalty. Goll (1979) contends that the child is the silent spokesperson for the family's distrust of the surrounding community. In other words, the parents' distrust of persons outside the family can become the model for the child's inhibition with strangers.

Sluzki (1983) observed the explicit rules of silence in the families of two nine-year-old female clients. In one of the families, the rules of silence were very explicit: "Whatever is not mentioned does not exist," while in the other family Sluzki reported "glimpses of rules of silence and of skeletons in the closet" that tend to support these rules. The notion of "skeletons in the closet" was based on the therapist's suspicion that the mother of the nine-year-old girl had been previously subjected to an incestuous relationship with the father.

The Krolian (1988) study indicates the importance of secrets in the development of elective mutism. The eight-year-old electively mute boy described a series of "ghosts in the closet" including "1000-year-old grandfather ghosts, 99-year-old father ghosts" and a variety of "kid ghosts." In this instance, however, it was the *therapist* who was instructed not to tell anyone in his family about them. In contrast to the child's keeping secrets within the family the scenario here seems to relate to keeping secrets from family members.

RULE-GOVERNED BEHAVIOR

Note[7.1]

Fear acquisition can occur, for example, through a child's being bullied or through self-generated negative thoughts and images. Fears are frequently connected with faulty family rules. Family rules are reflected in the "shoulds," "musts," "can'ts," and "oughts" in the verbal behavior of the client. For example, a child might learn that "It is okay to talk as long as what you say is correct." Another family rule which might be correlated with elective mutism is that you should not say anything which might annoy anyone. The rules become internalized and the client gradually comes to believe he avoids the anticipated negative consequences by refusing to speak. But as long as the client continues to experience the relief associated with electing to be silent, he is not able to be free from these dysfunctional family rules. The majority of therapies involve the client testing the validity of family rules. The client is empowered to recognize that he does not always have to agree with the family rules or that he does not always have to be correct in order to be accepted. Behavior therapists would probably refer to the above as dysfunctional rule-governed behavior.

Jackson (1965) wrote a seminal article entitled "Family Rules: Martial Quid Pro Quo."[1] Essential to Jackson's scheme is the concept of family rules – as the title clearly suggests. Jackson argued that behavior within the family depends as much upon the nature of the relationships as on the personality of the individuals who compose the relationships. Jackson's concept of "family rules" is an alternative to approaches which emphasize personality differences in relationships. Jackson offers a delightful example in support of his argument:

Imagine two perfectly identical persons – not real-life identical twins who have long since become distinguishable to themselves and others – but a carbon-copy pair who are in fact the same person in two bodies. If such a pair were to live together, it is obvious they would have to evolve differences which did not before exist. The first time they approached a door that must be entered in single file, the die would be cast. Who is to go first? On what basis is this decision to be made? After it is made and effected, can things ever be the same again? If they fight, someone must win. If one precedes and the other forbears, it cannot then be said they are identical, since one would be aggressive, thoughtless, or "the one who takes the initiative," while the other would be passive, patient, or sluggish. In short, a relationship problem which has nothing to do with individual differences – for there were none in our hypothetical pair – has been solved by evolving differences which may be considered shorthand expressions of the definition of the relationship which was achieved. Later, these differences are available to handle other, similar circumstances wherein identical simultaneous actions are neither possible nor desirable (p. 79).

Note the words "aggressive" and "thoughtless" which Jackson used to describe one of the people in the hypothetical relationship and the words "passive" and "patient" to describe the second person. The words "aggressive" and "thoughtless" are similar to the adjectives which might be used to describe Satir's "blamer" while the words "passive" and "patient" might be included among the adjectives used to describe the Satir's "placater" (Satir, 1972). According to Satir (1972), "Blamers" and "Placaters" are relationship types which correspond to specific verbal and non-verbal behaviors and often both are in the same family.

A later text (Bross, 1982) refers to the contribution of Jackson and defines family rules as follows:

Interaction among family members is not random. Over time, the full range of possible interaction sequences becomes restricted. Covert agreement arises concerning what categories of behaviour are acceptable or not and, moreover, the tolerable range of variation within acceptable categories. Consequently, interpersonal interaction comes increasingly to exhibit redundant interaction sequences. As inferred by an observer, such sequences are called "rules" (p. 57).

---

[1] Quid Pro Quo literally means "something for something" (Jackson, 1965, p. 80).

The notion of family rules within models of marital therapy may also be viewed within the more generic learning theory framework. If one observes "antecedent events – behavior – consequences" of family members, this undoubtedly leads one to formulate rules about "antecedent events – behavior – reinforcement" and "antecedent events – behavior – punishment." Repeatedly observing a family member being "angrily" yelled at for talking and the resultant silences of that person may enable the observer to formulate his or her own rule – in our example "being silent" terminates or avoids being "yelled at." In this illustration, the model which would account for the acquisition of the avoidance or escape response of "silence" is modeling. The major conditions necessary for modeling to occur are minimal and, therefore, it would not be difficult for one to learn the escape or avoidance response. One would only have to observe (attend to) the antecedent event – behavior – consequence, remember the three-fold sequence and execute the response of silence. My example seems to fit contingency-shaped behavior. In this instance, the contingency is learned via modeling – although the person could be a participant rather than an observer in the three-fold sequence. In the strict sense, however, rule-governed behavior often takes the form of a verbal or written statement which addresses each of the three components of the operant learning sequence. A child, for example, might hear one of his parents say, "If you talk when your mother and I are talking about something important you will be sent to your room." Here, "mother and father talking about something important" is the *antecedent event*, "if you talk" is an anticipated future *behavior*, and "you will be sent to your room" is the *consequence*.

Martin and Pear (1992) distinguish between contingency shaped and rule-governed behavior. They indicated that:

Contingency-shaped behavior is behavior that has been strengthened simply because it has been followed by reinforcement. No verbalizations, either overt or covert, are involved in strengthening or evoking the behavior. Rule-governed behavior, on the other hand, is behavior that is controlled by descriptions of the contingencies (i.e., the relationships) between specific responses and specific reinforcers. These descriptions of contingencies can act as stimuli that evoke appropriate behavior, providing that the individual has received reinforcement for emitting appropriate behavior in the presence of (or immediately after) these descriptions or rules (p. 45).

It seems clear from the above excerpt then that in rule-governed behavior, the consequences are speaker-mediated. A further critical analysis of rule-governed behavior is offered by Zettle and Hayes (1982). They claimed that:

Rules that specify the discriminative stimulus, the behavior, and the consequence may be more effective than our usual rules, which specify these components only vaguely; but the actual reinforcer for rule-following may not be the consequence that is specified in the rule. Furthermore, rule-following is an escape procedure. An implication is that the functional consequence is not the one specified in the rule, such as the good grades that will result from studying and doing homework assignments or the sound teeth that will result from flossing, or the bad grades that will result from not studying and not doing homework assignments or the cavities and tooth loss that will result from not flossing. Rather, the functional consequences may be a negative reinforcer; rule-following terminates self-blame, guilt, anxiety, or some other private event and thereby is reinforced (p. 35).

Rule use seems to qualify as operant behavior, however, because following or not following rules is subject to reinforcement and punishment. A rule, however, has no topography of its own. Worded another way, it would be difficult to envision what a "photograph" of "rule-following" behavior would look like. Indeed, how can an observer know that another person is using a rule? An inference is required but the inference is based on objective evidence.

Reese (1989) has offered six criteria for inferring rule use: (1) regularity of behavior is often used as evidence for behavior guided by rules. This criterion may be faulted, however, because behavior may be regular without being rule-governed. For example, a behavior may be regular because it was conditioned or instinctive but this has nothing to do with its being rule-governed, (2) continuous changes in behavior may be used as support for contingency-shaped behavior while discontinuous changes may be interpreted as rule-governed. The continuity-discontinuity issue refers to the degree to which prior experience influences present performance (continuity) or does not influence present performance (discontinuity), (3) the reported awareness of using a rule is often taken as evidence for inferring rule use. Indirect evidence of rule use may include the verbal reports of the user. A statement such as "I follow the rule because . . ." would be an obvious example of this type of self-report. Self-reports are based on indirect evidence rather than on direct observation. This feature is not unique to rule-governed behavior, however, because it applies to verbal reports about imagery, cognitions, sensations and other events which can not be seen by external observers, (4) if the person's behavior is observed to be consistent with a rule, then the use of the rule can be inferred, e.g., some teachers tell their students that they are required to participate in class discussions. This means that if one observed a student asking questions or spontaneously making comments we would be inclined to say that the verbal behavior of the person was consistent with the teacher's "participation rule," (5) a criterion for inferring rule use is concomitant behavior – that is, behavior that can be expected to accompany the use of a rule,[2] and (6) the strongest inference is based on the rule-generalization criterion. Evidence for this criterion is based on direct observation of the person or indirect evidence from the verbal reports of the person that the behavior occurs across different people, and settings. The comment by Berlyne (cited in Reese, 1989) may be helpful in clarifying the rule-generalization criterion. Berlyne claimed that:

If behavior is rule-governed (not his term), the behavior that represents the rule should be performed "with equal mastery" in all relevant situations, but if the behavior reflects "the acquisition of certain stimulus-response associations by direct learning and the emergence of other stimulus-response associations by stimulus-response generalization, then we should expect a generalization decrement, such as is found with stimulus generalization and with response generalization" (pp. 172–173).

---

[2] If I am required to give a ten-minute talk about a day in the life of my pet, then my taking photographs of my pet and keeping a one-day diary of the activities of my pet is consistent with the requirement of giving the brief talk. For this illustration, let us say that the notion of "requirement" is the equivalent of a "rule." The "rule" was that I give a ten-minute talk and I was observed to give a ten-minute talk. My behavior was not only consistent with the "rule" but the concomitant behaviors of "taking photographs" and "making diary entries" are evidence of my intent to permit my behavior be governed by the rule.

SELF-CONTROL THEORY

The self-control formulation which I am suggesting is based on the principles of operant conditioning. Electively mute individuals may learn the rule that "it's safer not to say anything because I might inadvertently tell on my parents" or "I might give the wrong answer and this would be personally embarrassing." The patient avoids these risks and adheres to the rule by using silence as a self-controlling response. Many of us have heard people say "I had better not say anything because once I start. . . ." Silence is also adopted by children as a self-controlling response for profane or obscene language. Elson *et al.* (1965) argue that elective mutism in some children is associated with the belief that speech is endowed with magical powers including the ability to inflict injury. The patient, therefore, reduces the likelihood of harming other people by becoming electively mute. Elson *et al.* also argue that the child protects loved ones by directing the silence to other individuals. According to the proposed self-control theory, the patient uses silence as a self-controlling response to inhibit inappropriate verbalizations. In this way, the patient not only controls the topography of the anger response (albeit inappropriately) but also avoids or minimizes the risk of punishment.

LANGUAGE-VOCAL DIFFERENCES THEORY

Scientist-practitioners have commented on the role of a peculiar accent or voice quality in the development of elective mutism. For example, an adolescent male may be embarrassed if he judges his voice to be effeminate or if others tell him that his voice is effeminate and tease him about it. In this case, speaking may be connected with verbal abuse and with negative nonverbal responses. As would be predicted from learning theory, speaking is reduced to avoid or escape ridicule.

I envision two phases for a language-vocal differences theory of elective mutism. Because the patient's language development is typically normal and because he speaks to certain individuals or in selected settings, it is hypothesized that escape responses precede avoidance behaviors. In the first phase, the patient uses silence to escape when he begins to receive negative consequences from others or as soon as he begins to experience self-generated unpleasant thoughts or negative physiological responses. Escape learning, therefore, is a likely explanation for the development of elective mutism. The second phase evolves when the patient avoids speaking in the situations in which he previously escaped from negative consequences by electing to be silent. In other words, it seems that avoidance learning is probably responsible for maintaining the silence user role. The specific characteristics of the two phases need to be studied.

Research

Bednar (1974), Bozigar and Hansen (1984), Bradley and Sloman (1975), Calhoun and Koenig (1973) and Conrad *et al.* (1974) found the incidence of elective mutism to be higher in bilingual children. Croghan and Craven (1982) speculate that the child may favor the deeply encoded language system and may therefore avoid speaking the second language. This may explain why some immigrant children do not speak at school. Similarly, Meyers (1984) said that immigrant children have a higher incidence of elective mutism because of the difficulty of learning a new language and the barriers to cultural adjustment.

HOSTILITY THEORY

Wahlroos (1974) in *Family Communication* discusses how the nonverbal behavior of silence can be used as a weapon. The person may discover that prolonged silences trouble other people. Not all prolonged silences are expressions of hostility but the communication context assists the silence receiver in labeling the prolonged silence as a hostile response. The discomfort of others may reinforce the use of prolonged silence and silence may become a preferred mode of expressing hostility. I contend that instrumental learning is operating in at least three ways. First, the individual is able to express disagreement or anger in a potent way while simultaneously reducing the risk of punishment. This passive expression of hostility reduces the unpleasant consequences which are frequently associated with responses of physical aggression or verbal abuse. Second, the person is positively reinforced by the visible discomfort of others. Third, the patient may receive additional unintended positive reinforcement. In non-behavioral terminology this is called secondary gain. In the context of the proposed hostility theory, secondary gain implies that in addition to safely expressing anger, the patient receives other "advantages." These positive "side effects" are frequently associated with the attempts of others to get the patient to talk. Because this may be one of the only times that the patient receives attention, family members and friends may be inadvertently reinforcing the inappropriate use of silence.

Research

Hayden (1980) included passive-aggressive mutism in his classification of elective mutism. The use of silence was viewed as a "weapon." Parker *et al.* (1960) described the fathers of their patients as passive, inactive socially, and non-speaking when angry. This description suggests that the fathers employ the silence-user role in expressing disagreement or anger. Rosenberg and Lindblad (1978) also indicated that the patient's unadaptive use of silence is a passive-aggressive maneuver. In addition, the elective mute may even equate speaking with "giving in" (Wilkins, 1985).

INTEGRATION THEORY

Sluzki (1983) argues that under certain circumstances, the symptom picture of elective mutism serves an integrative function. This researcher's interpretation is reflected in the following excerpt:

The therapist . . . told the 9-year-old girl that he was moved by the sacrifice of silence she made to bear witness to her daddy that she was not betraying him by speaking the language of a country that brought him so much bitterness and disappointment, while bearing witness to her mommy that she did not betray her and thus went to school and learned all the many things offered by a country that was so generous and kind to her (pp. 73–74).

Here, the integrative function of elective mutism is a response to cultural conflict rather than the expression or inhibition of anger.

CHAPTER 8

FEIGNING THE SILENCE USER ROLE

INTRODUCTION

Malingering is the feigning of disease (Rogers, 1989a, b). It is a product of a society which provides compensation for those who are sick or disabled. Resnick (1989) cautions that there are certain conditions which at first impression appear like malingering.

Partial malingering is the conscious exaggeration of existing symptoms or the fraudulent allegation that prior genuine symptoms are still present. In addition, the term false imputation refers to the ascribing of actual symptoms to a cause consciously recognized to have no relationship to the symptoms. . . . In addition to conscious deception, some individuals mistakenly believe that there is a relationship between an accident and their psychological or physical disability. These patients may fail to realize that consecutive events do not necessarily have a causal relationship. Such genuine misperceptions should be differentiated from conscious attempts at deception (Resnick, 1989, p. 85).

The feigning of a specific symptom is a voluntary action of the person. The concept of malingered elective mutism, therefore, is troublesome because a diagnosis of "elective mutism" indicates that the use of silence is *voluntary*. Furthermore, symptom relief such as fear reduction and secondary gain associated with, for example, being able to control the behavior of others is often attributed to the clinical picture of elective mutism (Reed, 1963).

INCONSISTENT RESPONDING

Malingering has often been detected by noting inconsistencies in the patient's verbal statements within and between interviews. The assumption is that if the patient can respond appropriately at one time during the assessment, his or her failure to respond appropriately at another time is evidence for malingering. In the case of mutism, one might expect to observe consistency in the person's use of silence. Observations of suspected elective mutism should therefore reveal that (1) the person is consistently silent in the target setting and (2) the individual consistently speaks in a setting or settings outside the target location.

OVERPLAYING THE MALINGERED RESPONSE

The "overplay" approach assumes that malingerers who are naive to elective mutism will "overplay" the role so that their malingered use of silence does not resemble true elective mutism. The "overplay" approach, however, seems unsuitable for detecting malingered elective mutism because the verbal production of the electively mute person is typically zero or near zero. A closer examination of this issue, however, is required. An electively mute child or adolescent may speak in the non-speaking setting *if a person he or she speaks to outside of the setting is present.* Therefore, in this scenario, individuals who are feigning elective mutism would be predicted to overplay the silence user role so that they would be observed not to converse with the people that they speak to even if they were present in the non-speaking setting.

MALINGERING AND DEFENSIVENESS

The person who deliberately attempts to avoid disclosing a behavior problem or physical illness is described as responding defensively. In taking a psychological test, a person exhibiting a defensive reaction would avoid checking items which indicated pathology. Indeed, the person might endorse test items which would put him or her in a favorable light to get or keep a job. The malingerer, on the other hand, would check items indicating pathology in order to be released from employment or some other responsibility. Persons in trouble with the law may endorse items such as mutism if they believed that this would make them unsuitable to stand trial (Green, 1989).

Children and adolescents absent themselves verbally, but they do not absent themselves physically from the setting in which they elect to be silent. Furthermore, electively mute school-age persons often complete the required written work. Hence, persons suspected of being voluntarily mute could be interviewed provided they were given a choice of writing their responses, checking response options from a checklist or pointing to response alternatives in a multiple choice format. The "checking" and "pointing" options would be of limited usefulness because the "unknowns" about a crime would make it difficult to prepare the interview questions and the response options. The checklist method and the multiple choice approach is useful, however, in soliciting basic information such as place of residence. If the client responded to these types of questions, this would suggest that he or she could communicate in a mode other than verbal behavior. *According to the overplay hypothesis, the person who failed to check or point to response options or who refused to write answers to interview questions might be suspected of malingered mutism – especially if there was evidence based on direct observation that he or she could emit these responses in other settings.*

FEIGNING A BEHAVIORAL DEFICIT

Malingered elective mutism involves feigning a behavioral deficit rather than a behavioral excess. Thus, to fake elective mutism one only has to use silence consistently and for longer durations than one ordinarily does.

DECEPTION IN CHILDREN

Note[8.1]

Because elective mutism is primarily a disorder of childhood and adolescence, it is important for the clinician to be able to assess deception in children. Quinn (1988) has provided useful criteria for assessing deception in children. These guidelines may be helpful in detecting the deception of malingered elective mutism.

1. Does the child have the developmental capacity to deceive? The very young child's statements may be untruths generated by their immature cognitive abilities with no intention to deceive. As a general guideline, children under the age of 6 have been shown to be unable to lie successfully.

2. Does the child or adolescent have a history of persistent lying? If yes, is it possible that this admission is also a lie? This is often a complex area in the assessment of deception since even severely conduct-disordered youth may be telling the truth concerning the clinical or legal issue under investigation.

3. Does the child have a psychiatric disorder which would alter reality testing or cause severe distortion, fantasy, or use of defenses such as massive denial or dissociation? A seriously emotionally disturbed child may make statements which are not lies but rather a product of a mental disorder. Such distortions may include the psychotic adolescent who makes an allegation of sexual abuse against a nurse, despite the presence of witnesses who can attest that no abuse was observed on the occasion in question, or the borderline child who sexualizes interactions. Clinicians should be well informed concerning developmental norms of cognition and the individual child's history, including sexual history, in order to fully investigate complaints.

4. Is there a psychosocial stressor which may promote lying? A careful evaluation should elicit the effect of divorce, or other aspects of family life, on the child. Equally important is the assessment of how the child is coping with psychosocial stressors and what pressures

are experienced, either to dramatize the situation or minimize the family conflict.

5. Has the child's deception guilt decreased? Has the child's deception apprehension increased? The clinician should seek to understand the child's beliefs about his or her own statements and whether these beliefs cause the child to have increased or decreased secondary guilt or anxiety which confound the clinical assessment.

6. Is the child pursuing a nonmoral objective? For example, is the child seeking to remain with one parent by bringing an allegation against the other? The clinician should attempt to understand the goal being pursued by the child and how the child believes his or her statements aid in pursuit of the goal.

7. Is an adult lying for the child or distorting the child's communication? Examples may include the conscious deception or overinterpretation by parents in custody and visitation battles or the rare phenomenon of Munchausen syndrome by proxy . . . in which there is a parental falsification of medical illness in children.

8. Is the child's presentation of a psychiatric or medical disorder consistent with a well-recognized illness or syndrome? A clinician should consider malingering, factitious illness, atypical symptomatology, conversion disorder, as well as the somatoform disorders, as differential diagnoses.

9. Does this or previous mental health assessments contain interviewing errors resulting in incorrect assessment of the nature of the child's communication? For example, highly coercive and leading questioning by an interviewer may lead to the premature conclusion that sexual abuse has occurred (pp. 115–117).

A student who was observed not to speak in the classroom for over a year, for example, would be electively mute according to DSM–III–R and DSM–IV Options. If students wish to present a favorable impression to their parents, for example, they might claim that they do talk in the class, do answer the teacher's questions and do volunteer to answer questions, when direct observation shows that they do not do any of these things. This response profile would be both deceptive and defensive. Such a response pattern from an electively mute child might even be consistent with the parental belief that their child does talk in the classroom, and with disbelief when they are informed that he or she does not talk in class. The parents' reaction is understandable, however, because electively mute children ordinarily speak to family members in the home. The client's deceptive and defensive responses about speaking in class do not indicate malingered mutism; they only suggest that for whatever reason the person wishes to conceal from his or her parents the fact that he or she does not talk in class. The astute clinician would, however, attempt to account for the deception.

LEGAL ASPECTS OF ELECTIVE MUTISM

According to Daniel and Resnick (1987) to be perceived mentally ill is to be found unsuitable to stand trial and this enables the person to avoid punishment. Refusing to speak for a prolonged time is not an easy sacrifice and would not be predicted to occur unless an individual is facing a severe penalty. Few people can go without speaking for more than a few minutes let alone for long periods of time because the silence user role involves (1) remaining silent in the face of statements which ought to be contradicted or denied; (2) denying oneself companionship; (3) rejecting offers of friendship; and (4) refusing to ask for luxuries to which one may have been accustomed (Davidson cited in Daniel and Resnick, 1987).

Daniel and Resnick (1987) did not refer to elective mutism or to standard nomenclatures such as DSM–III–R. DSM–III–R guidelines indicate that the person speaks in certain circumstances and does not speak in at least one location or situation. The essential question is whether or not an electively mute individual is competent to stand trial especially when such a person is *unwilling rather than unable to talk.* According to Daniel and Resnick pentothal interviews might uncover the true nature of the mutism and observing the individuals at unexpected times in the settings in which they elect not to talk might reveal that they can and do talk.

The role of trauma in the onset of elective mutism is discussed in Chapter 7. The elective mutism literature and the standard nomenclatures do not mention any restrictions on the type of trauma which may lead to elective mutism. Indeed, the literature on elective mutism concedes that there are conditions which are correlated with the onset and maintenance of elective mutism. One such circumstance could be the psychological trauma associated with arrest for a serious offence and the likelihood of conviction and severe punishment. In the case of criminal behavior, the trauma probably coincides with the arrest, the likelihood of conviction, and the anticipated severity of the sentence. These events not only seem to fit the trauma hypothesis but, in addition, the trauma associated with criminal behavior is as severe as many of the events which have been correlated with the onset of elective mutism.

In the typical case of elective mutism the client escapes or avoids an unpleasant situation by electing to be silent. *In many instances, others go along with the silence and consequently there is often a delay between observing the problem and referring the individual for assessment and treatment.* This means that in the majority of the cases of elective mutism, the escape or avoidance of real or anticipated events occur *before the client has been officially diagnosed electively mute*. The reverse, however, seems to be the case for individuals who are suspected of being unsuitable to stand trial by virtue of mutism because escape or avoidance does not solely depend on the mutistic behavior but on a psychiatric examination and securing the psychiatric label of elective mutism.

If the accused person received bail while awaiting trial, the diagnostic guidelines for elective mutism would predict that the accused person would talk in settings other than those associated with the criminal justice system. To the police and solicitors who are unfamiliar with elective mutism, this could readily indicate malingering while, in fact, the silence user would be exhibiting a typical pattern of elective mutism as specified in DSM–III–R, DSM–IV Options and in the mental health literature.

The critical issue, as emphasized by Daniel and Resnick (1987), is whether or not the mutism is under the defendant's voluntary control. The very term "elective mutism" suggests, however, that the mutism is under voluntary control. DSM–III–R or DSM–IV Options do not address the voluntariness or involuntariness of the mutistic response and, therefore, these recognized diagnostic sources are not useful in clarifying this issue. Once the mutism is established, the individual predictably speaks in identified stimulus conditions and predictably does not speak in at least one other identified setting. The above discussion, therefore, raises important questions about the usefulness of the term malingered mutism because the term "elective mutism" indicates that the use of silence is voluntary as is malingered mutism.

MALINGERING

Escape and avoidance occurs in a number of behavior disorders including elective mutism. For example, the school phobic expresses his fear by refusing to enter the school setting while the electively mute person will go into the setting but will not speak. I have yet to see elective mutism referred to as malingering, and investigators who have asked the individuals at the conclusion of treatment why they elected to be silence users have found no support for malingering. Perhaps the notion of malingering has been dismissed because (1) the electively mute person is *consistently silent* in the target setting and (2) the person has been frequently observed to be electively mute for in excess of six months in the target setting.

The incidence of elective mutism among adults is almost negligible. Since elective mutism is extremely rare among adults, a statistical notion of an extremely low probability of adult elective mutism might be used as an argument in support of malingering among adults who are brought before the courts. I seriously question the validity of such a position, however, because although elective mutism is extremely rare among adults we should not preclude the occurrence of the "unique case."

RELATIVE PUNISHMENTS FOR SPEAKING AND ELECTING TO BE SILENT

Once an individual becomes accustomed to a setting, he or she can readily identify the behaviors which are sanctioned and the responses which are likely to be punished. In the classroom, for example, silence meets with the teacher's approval while unauthorized talking may be punished. Children also become aware of the relative rewards and punishments for being silent and for talking. One might suspect that there are greater rewards for being silent than for talking. Similarly, one might also conjecture that the punishments for being silent in one setting are less severe than the punishments for talking. These circumstances may account for the fact that the setting for the silence in the majority of cases of elective mutism is the classroom. It seems reasonable to also suggest that a teacher is less inconvenienced by the excessively silent student than by the excessively talkative student. If this proposition is correct, it may account for the delay between a teacher's observing the mutism and referring the child for treatment.

For adults, however, who are accustomed to using verbal behavior to ask for what they want, I believe that the reverse is true. In addition to the advantages of talking discussed by Daniel and Resnick (1987), there are others which are so natural that we rarely think of them. Adults have learned that the support obtained through talking with others can lessen the impact of negative consequences. Asking for clarification or for information often leads to substituting healthy ways of thinking and acting for unhealthy ways of thinking and acting. Verbal exchange can also help to maintain behavior during the delay between setting and achieving a goal.

CHILD-ADOLESCENT ELECTIVE MUTISM

Adults would find it difficult to meet their needs and wants without the medium of verbal behavior. Children have been accustomed to having many of their needs and wants met without depending on verbal behavior while the reverse is true for adults. It is not surprising, therefore, that *the incidence of elective mutism decreases rapidly with increasing age*. Table 8.1 presents additional information based on the published literature which may have implications for the elective mutism – malingering issue.

Malingering would be predicted to occur in response to an identifiable

Table 8.1. Child and adolescent elective mutism.

Variable	Comment
Trauma	Coincides with an identifiable trauma
Sex	Occurs primarily in females
Criminal behavior	Absence of published studies relating elective mutism to criminal behavior
Escape and avoidance	Official labeling not required for child or adolescent to escape or avoid aversive stimuli through the silence user role. For a person accused of a criminal offence silence user behavior permits escape or avoidance only if the person is officially labeled electively mute.
Malingering	Closest reference to malingering is Reed's "attention-getting – manipulative elective mutism"
Referral	Delay of approximately six months to two years. If malingered mutism is suspected, immediate assessment is required to determine suitability to stand trial.

trauma which could include fear of arrest, being charged, or of conviction and the anticipated punishment severity. Trauma, however, is also correlated with the onset of elective mutism, and hence this criterion cannot be used to distinguish between elective mutism and malingering. In addition, there are no clinical reports in the literature relating criminal behavior to elective mutism.

Because of the typical delay in being referred for assessment, the child or adolescent has an opportunity to use silence to escape or avoid negative events for a longer time than an accused individual who elects to become a silence user to escape or avoid the negative consequences of the judicial system. *This means that the sooner the accused person is officially labelled electively mute, the sooner he can use silence as an escape or avoidance response.* The silence user role enables the child to "avoid" or "escape" but an adult who is accused of committing a criminal offence must become a silence user and, in addition, be officially diagnosed as electively mute.

The silence user on being labelled electively mute, need not, however, be deemed unsuitable to stand trial. Although an audio recording would be unsuitable, other methods could be used to record the proceedings. For example, the accused individual could write his responses to questions even though it may be slow and tedious. This parallels what happens to electively mute children in school. Often, electively mute children perform rather well in all activities except those requiring speech. The electively mute child attends school and is expected to participate and do the same written work as the other students.

Similarly, if the accused persons understand the questions and discussions, they should be permitted to communicate in a modality other than verbal behavior. Perhaps such individuals could be instructed to write their responses and, where feasible, to respond by using gestures to indicate "yes" or "no." This would mean that the transcription of proceedings would have to include written statements and nonverbal responses such as agreed-upon gestures. In this instance, a videotape recording would be the appropriate transcription method. To judge a person who has good receptive language unable to stand trial on the basis of the absence of verbal behavior suggests that only the verbal modality is suitable for a person to participate in court proceedings. If this is the case, this suggests an unnecessarily rigid and restrictive judicial system.

CHAPTER 9

DIRECT OBSERVATION OF BEHAVIOR

MOLAR AND MOLECULAR DESCRIPTION

The following illustration will be used in distinguishing between molar and molecular description.

Molecular description		Molar description
Movements of the lips, tongue, facial muscles, arms, legs, trunk and diaphragm.	versus	Oral presentation to class

The description of behavior on the right involves the person; those on the left involve *independent parts of the individual*. Molar behavior is goal directed. An action always involves "getting to" or "getting from" something or someone. Molar behavior occurs within the cognitive field of the person. This means that people emitting the behavior know what they are doing and can describe their behavior through the medium of language.

Molecular description was used in the Subak *et al.* (1982) study. The authors reported that the adolescent responded to questions by nodding her head or shrugging her shoulders. In addition, she was skilled at expressing her different moods by slightly changing the position of her lips or eyebrows.

INTERPRETATIONS

Interpretations frequently involve statements about behaviors or situations rather than statements which are based on the principles and theories of human behavior. When interpretations are used, they are set apart in an indented paragraph so that they can be studied. The following example illustrates an interpretation about behavior followed by a description of behavior and setting.

[In answering the teacher's questions, the children seemed worried and frightened.]

Whenever a student gave the wrong answer the teacher raised his voice, came over to the student's desk and yelled, "You never can do anything right; I have never heard of such a stupid answer."

Interpretations involving statements about behavior are useful because they identify the context of behavior.

The second type of interpretation is based on *theories about behavior*. As with interpretations involving statements about behavior, observers should identify interpretations based on theory and research. Interpretations should be based on recorded observations.

IDENTIFYING BEHAVIORAL EPISODES

The primary characteristic of an episode is consistency in the direction of the behavior. To episode, according to Wright (1967), is "to find boundaries between parts of a behavior sequence" (p. 65). A change in episode occurs when there is a change in the direction of behavior. Wright indicated that the following cues are associated with the beginning and ending of episodes:

1. Change in the "sphere" of the behavior from verbal to physical to social to intellectual, or from any of these to another.
2. Change in the part of the body predominantly involved in a physical action, as from hand to mouth to feet.
3. Change in the physical direction of the behavior. Now a child is walking north to a sandpile; next, he is going up a tree; later, he climbs down the tree.
4. Change in behavior object . . . as from a knife to a watch to a dog to a person.
5. Change in the present behavior setting. When his teacher says, "Pass," Henry leaves the classroom setting and, at the same time, starts a new action.
6. Change in the tempo of activity, as when a child shifts from walking leisurely to running toward a friend (p. 68).

Episoding involves identifying the goal of the behavior and identifying if the behavior brings the person nearer to the goal. The following example identifies these two processes:

Wesley Mead, in a darkened room, turns on a light. Then he goes at once to a wall and stands before it, looking at the picture. Is *Turning on Light* a separate episode or is it only the first phase of a large episode, *Looking at Picture?* This question can only be answered by finding whether or not, in turning on the light, Wesley intended to view the picture (Wright, 1967, p. 75).

A second example shows the importance of considering change in the direction of behavior.

[The] six-year-old who has been ordered sternly by his mother to stay at home first runs off to the school playground and then goes to the house of a friend. We probably could mark *Running to School Playground* and *Going to House of a Friend* as separate episodes on the ground that the two actions differ in direction (Wright, 1967, p. 77).

An episode includes not only the behavior involved in getting to a goal but also the behavior that is associated with reaching the goal.

According to Wright (1967) "interruption is defined as a drop in potency of an episode to zero before the person has reached the goal" (p. 90). Suppose that a colleague comes to my office while I am grading papers. I stop briefly to talk and then resume grading the papers immediately after she leaves. Wright would argue for one rather than two episodes because after the interruption I resumed my activity.

TYPES OF EPISODES

Overlapping occurs when episodes occur, wholly or in part, at one time. Wright (1967) identified three types of episodes: the coinciding, the enclosing – enclosed and the interlinking. The attributes of these episodes are presented in Fig. 9.1.

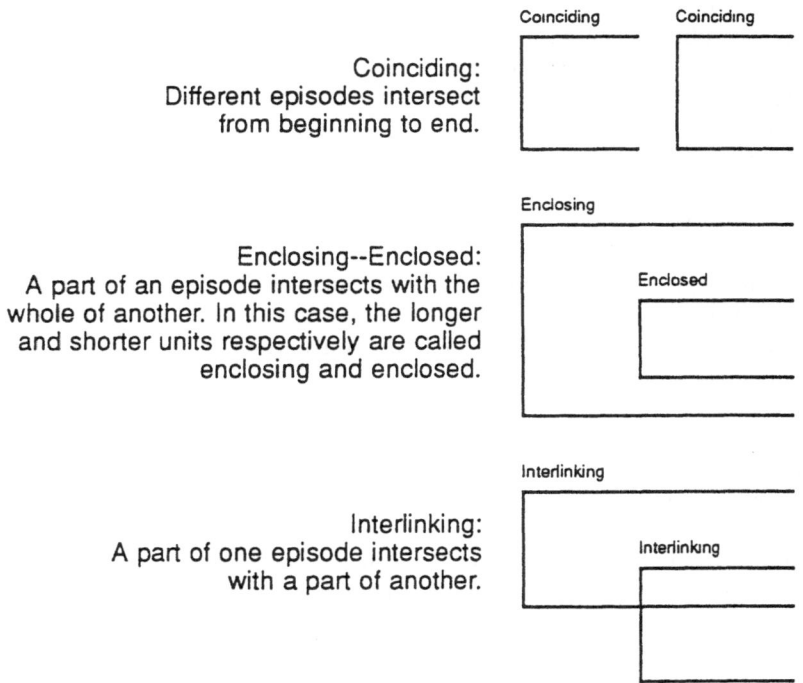

Coinciding:
Different episodes intersect
from beginning to end.

Enclosing--Enclosed:
A part of an episode intersects with the whole of another. In this case, the longer and shorter units respectively are called enclosing and enclosed.

Interlinking:
A part of one episode intersects
with a part of another.

Note: Adapted from Fig. 4.1. Different types of episode overlap. Wright, H.F. (1967). *Recording and Analyzing Child Behavior.* New York: Harper & Row.

Fig. 9.1. Coinciding, enclosing-enclosed, and interlinking behavioral episodes.

REPORTING OBSERVATIONS

The observer should report as fully as possible the context and behavior of the subject. The description of the setting should include the main characters, their positions, and the main features of the physical setting. For example, if a child is drawing a picture and is oblivious to the activity of other children, it is important to report this observation because one might ordinarily expect the other children to elicit a response from the child. Because this is an interpretation about behavior, it is important to set the interpretation apart in an indented paragraph. If a child draws a picture, the observer should describe the picture and report the reactions of the child to the picture and the responses of the other people.

It is important to provide a clear description of the *sequence of the behaviour and to observe for a long enough duration to make sense out of the observations.* I observed a student preparing a bulletin board for a class assignment. The student had a white cylinder secured between her chin and neck. My initial impression was that the cylinder was a type of prosthetic device related to a neck injury. I later observed the student holding a white cardboard can with her left hand while taking red poster tacks out of the can with her right hand to affix a picture to the bulletin board. Observing for a long enough duration enabled me to make an accurate observation – namely, that the "prosthetic device" was actually a can that the student held under her chin, which enabled her to position the picture with one hand and to affix the picture with the other.

The observer should describe the behaviors which occurred rather than behaviors which did not occur. For example, the statement, "The child maintained eye contact" is preferred to the statement "The child did not look away." The negative reporting of observations lacks the precision of positively reporting behaviour. One knows only what the subject did not do; one does not have a picture of the behavior of the person.

The guidelines for writing reports of observations are primarily concerned with the method of specimen description, but they are useful for writing even the most rudimentary reports. The observer should take notes in the observation setting and record the observations on an audiotape immediately after making the observations. After this is done, Wright (1967) recommends that another person listen to the tape who has not observed the behavior. The role of this person is to identify the parts of the specimen records which are unclear or incomplete and to ask the observer for clarification (Wright, 1967). An accurate record of observations enables a person who has not observed the behavior to model the movements of the individual's body parts (molecular behavior) as well as the movements of the whole person (molar responses).

The observer should record his or her observations immediately after each observation session. Every effort should be made to avoid writing retrospective reports. The greater the time interval between making the observations and writing the report of the observations, the greater the likelihood will be that the report will resemble a retrospective report. A retrospective report is based on information about the past obtained now. Robins (1966), in *Deviant Children Grow Up*, claims that one of the problems of retrospective reporting is that what is reported frequently depends on the outcome of the problem event. According to Robins, if the outcome was positive, the past behavior and circumstances will be reported as being more positive than if the outcome was negative. When there is substantial time between making the observations and writing the report there is also the temptation to substitute interpretations of behavior for descriptions of behavior by altering the description to match the outcome. When my students write reports based on direct observation, I ask them to indicate the date of the observations and the date of the report. The readers can then draw their own conclusions about the accuracy of the record of the observations. A short interval (such as a couple of days) between making the observations and writing the report probably indicates greater accuracy than a delay of several weeks.

CHAPTER 10

SCATTER PLOT:
APPLICATIONS FOR ELECTIVE MUTISM

INTRODUCTION

The scatter plot technique described by Touchette *et al.* (1985) is useful in identifying patterns of speaking and suggests environmental features that occasion the use of silence. According to Touchette *et al.* the technique is especially helpful in depicting short episodes of responding alternating with periods of no responding. Even severe behavior problems do not occur at a steady rate. Instead, there are periods of high response and others of no response during the course of a day. The line graph method of displaying response frequency does not show the pattern of responding and therefore important changes within each day are not identified.

SCATTER PLOT CONSTRUCTION

The first step is to construct a grid similar to Fig. 10.2. Vertically, the grid divides time of day into hours, half hours, quarter hours, or any time unit appropriate to observing the client's speaking and electively mute behavior. The horizontal segments of the grid represent successive days.

SCATTER PLOT DATA

The data for scatter plots are frequency counts in half-hour or shorter observation intervals. Minimal training is needed and the simplicity of this method enables the observer to record directly on the scatter chart without performing any calculations.

INTEROBSERVER AGREEMENT

Touchette *et al.* (1985) used the following formula in calculating the agreement between two independent observers.

$$\frac{\text{agreements} \times 100}{\text{agreements} + \text{disagreements}}$$

An interval on the scatter plot is scored as agreement if both observers recorded the behavior as having occurred or not occurred at the same time.

CHARTING

A blank cell is used to represent a zero occurrence of the behavior and filled cells indicate that the behavior occurred during the interval. It is useful, however, to divide the occurrence category into high and low rates. The lower frequency can be recorded as a slash. More than three categories, however, produce charts that are difficult to interpret. The difference in frequency among the cells of the scatter plot identifies the pattern of the elective mutism. The scatter plot is a very flexible technique, but a grid must be selected so that the display is accurate and easily interpreted.

VISUAL ANALYSIS OF SCATTER PLOT DATA

A scatter plot can display periods during which the behavior problem almost never occurs or occurs with near certainty. The need for a scatter plot arises when the target behavior is frequent, and informal observations do not suggest a reliable correspondence with anything in particular. Electively mute behavior may be highly correlated with a time of day, the presence or absence of certain people, a social setting, a class of activities, a contingency of reinforcement, a physical environment, or a combination of these variables. The scatter plot facilitates the identification of a relationship between electively mute behavior and one or more environmental characteristics. Uninterpretable scatter plot data may reflect an unstable environment. For example, if a teacher is ill and a series of different teachers substitute in her place, frequency of responding cannot be tied to people. In unstable environments, the time of day in which the behavior occurs may be the only observable pattern.

In the case of elective mutism, Fig. 10.1 shows the number of words which were spoken by an electively mute child for five consecutive days. The graph reveals that the child spoke between 0–10 words per day in a target setting during the first five days of treatment. The visual representation, however, obscures the circumstances surrounding speaking episodes. In contrast, the scatter plot depicted in Fig. 10.2 indicates that speaking episodes occurred during three 30-minute observation intervals, specifically between 10:00–10:30 and 11:30–12:00 in the morning and between 2:30–3:00 in the afternoon.

The therapist is alerted to the specific circumstances of these speaking episodes such as the people present, activity of the speaker, and details of the physical setting which coincided with speaking. The line graph does

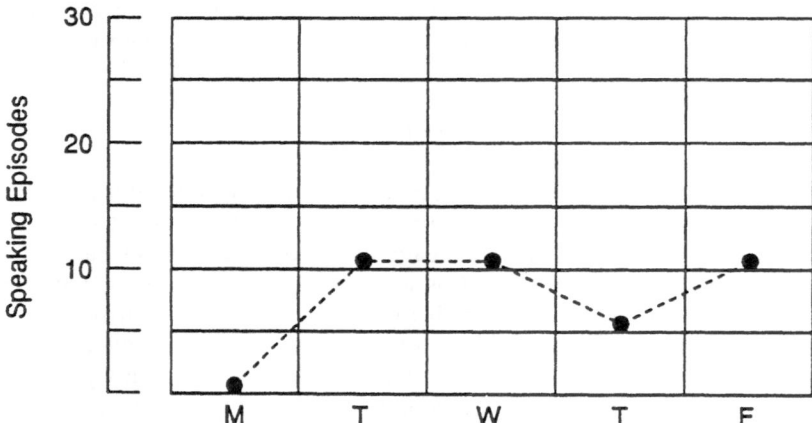

Fig. 10.1. Frequency chart of speaking episodes.

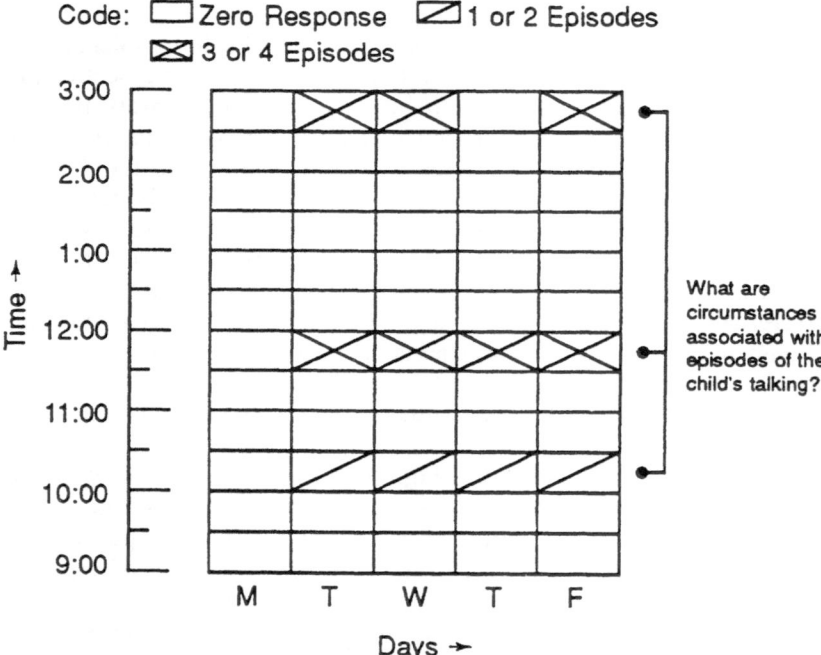

Fig. 10.2. Scatter plot of speaking episodes.

not permit the identification of these potentially important connections. The absence of speech on Thursday afternoon between 2:30–3:00 breaks the pattern of the other four days. By visually inspecting the scatter plot the therapist can explore the circumstances associated with the presence and absence of speaking.

SELF-MONITORING PRODUCED REACTIVE EFFECTS

Electively mute children could observe and record their own speaking episodes. This approach maximizes reactive effects which means that the potential for generating change is more likely to come from self-observation and self-recording than from monitoring and recording by external observers.

OBSERVING THE TARGET BEHAVIOR IN ANOTHER PERSON

There is another type of reactive effect which occurs when the person with the problem observes the same behavior in another person. For example, an electively mute child could be asked to observe and record speaking episodes of a peer. Having an electively mute person observe another person's behavior has several advantages. First, the focus is on monitoring speaking rather than silence and this is important because one of the major treatment goals is eliciting speech. Second, having an electively mute individual serve as an external observer would also be a useful training experience for later self-observation and self-recording. Third, monitoring the behavior of another person focuses on speaking without the threat of having to speak. Fourth, this approach gives the clinician an opportunity to positively reinforce children for observing and recording talking episodes.

A mediator could also be instructed to praise the speaking episodes of the peer that the electively mute child is observing. This would insure that positive consequences followed the peer's speaking and, in observing this pattern, the electively mute child would have an opportunity to discover the relationship between the peer's talking and positive consequences – and perhaps what would happen if he or she participated in class activities requiring a verbal response.

DISCUSSION

Although there are no published reports which have used the scatter plot to assess the behavior of elective mutism, the technique offers useful possibilities. One of the major features of elective mutism is that the child can and does talk in certain circumstances and, therefore, the technique should permit an observer to identify his or her specific pattern of talking.

The scatter plot has the advantage of permitting clinicians to (1) prepare
a more comprehensive assessment of the problem than would be permitted
by a line graph or informal methods of observation; (2) identify if verbal
responding is related to specific activities and people in the target setting;
(3) suggest guidelines for programming generalization of the target response;
(4) identify variations in verbal responding within and between days; and
(5) assess problem severity. For example, a child who spoke to a few people
during several learning activities would have a problem of lesser severity
than a child who rarely spoke during a variety of classroom activities.

TREATMENT PLANNING

The scatter plot permits the clinician to identify the settings and circumstances associated with the client's speaking. Furthermore, observers could
chart the location and number of speaking episodes during baseline and
treatment. This information, derived from the scatter plot, is useful in
assessing the effectiveness of interventions and in pinpointing planned-for
and unprogrammed generalizations of verbal responding. The scatter plot
would permit the clinician to modify the intervention if it indicated minimal
or no change in behavior.

During baseline, the scatter plot on the left in Fig. 10.3 indicates that
the child did not talk in any of the activities or to anyone between the

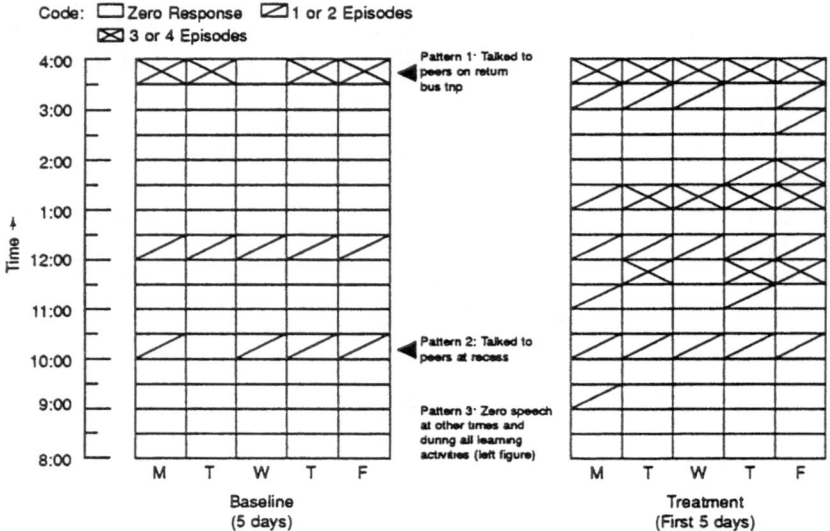

Fig. 10.3. Scatter plot for speaking episodes for baseline phase and treatment phase.

beginning of school in the morning until recess. During recess he was observed to talk to different children in a variety of play activities. The same pattern of responding applies to the noon recess and the pattern of silence for the afternoon was identical to that of the morning. Because the child did not speak to anyone during classroom activities, the problem might be described as severe but limited to school hours.

The child was observed to speak during free time at recess, during the lunch break, and during the half hour bus trip on the way home. What did the scatter plot reveal that the teacher did not already know? First, the scatter plot data may have confirmed the teacher's suspicions about the severity of the problem. Second, the scatter plot indicated that the reports which she received were only partly accurate. The children said that the child talked while on the bus. The precision of the scatter plot observations indicated that the child talked to the other children on the return trip in the afternoon but not during the trips to school on each of the five mornings of the baseline period.

In contrast to the baseline, the charted data for the treatment phase (right chart of Fig. 10.3) indicates that the intervention was effective on the first day of treatment. There were more speaking episodes and number of words spoken on the first day of treatment than on the last day of baseline.

Recording Multiple Behaviors: Multiple Cell Scatter Plot Technique

Employing a scatter plot in the setting in which the client speaks and in the setting in which he or she elects to be silent provides a comprehensive assessment of the target problem. Physically separating the scatter plot into the settings in which the client speaks and does not speak facilitates the visual inspection of the data. The original version of the scatter plot (Touchette et al., 1985) provided for the assessment of the frequency of one target behavior. I have found that in treating elective mutism, the person progresses from elective mutism to reluctant speech (e.g., responding when asked a question) to spontaneous or self-initiated speech.

One code is required for the frequency of the target responses such as ☐ zero response, ◲ for one or two responses and ⊠ for three or four responses. In order to record the occurrence of multiple types of speech (e.g., reluctant and spontaneous speech), two codes are required. For example, the notation "R" inside a cell indicates reluctant speech and the notation "S" indicates spontaneous speech. The symbol ◲ is used to record one or two occurrences of reluctant speech while the symbol ◲ is used to record one or two occurrences of self-initiated speech. The modified scatter plot means that each cell in which the occurrence of verbal behavior is indicated contains information about the type of behavior and the frequency of its occurrence. It may be necessary, however, to reduce the length of the observation intervals. This is because the shorter the observation interval, the less likely it will be that different types of speech will occur within the same cell.

Toward the end of a treatment for elective mutism, one might expect a single cell to contain both reluctant and spontaneous speech due to the greater frequency of each behavior. For example, the client might respond to a question and then ask a question of his or her own or he or she may volunteer information. In this instance, even short observation intervals would be inappropriate. Therefore, I recommend double cells for each observational interval (see Fig. 10.4).

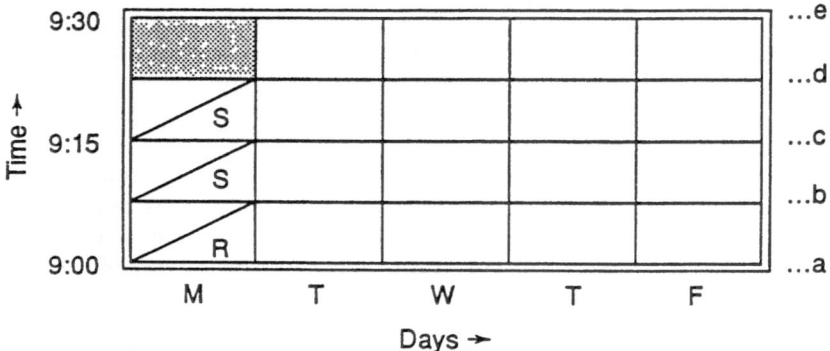

Fig. 10.4. Double entry scatter plot.

Reading across successive days, the double cells for the observation interval 9:00–9:15 are a–b and b–c. The double cells for 9:15–9:30 are c–d and d–e. For the observational interval between 9:00–9:15, one observes occurrences of reluctant and spontaneous speech. On Monday, reluctant speech occurred at least once between 9:00–9:15 and self-initiated speech also occurred at least once during the same time interval. The scatter plot also reveals the type and frequency of verbal behavior that occurred between 9:15–9:30 on Monday. The second set of cells (c–d and d–e) indicates two episodes of spontaneous speech. Since only one type of verbal response occurred between 9:15–9:30, only one of the two cells for this interval is used. The unused cell should be shaded to show that it an *unused cell* rather than a cell indicating the absence of verbal behavior.

DISCUSSION

Frequently, in the early stages of successful treatment, the electively mute person will respond to questions but will not ask a question or initiate other types of verbal responses. One must be cautious, therefore, in interpreting occurrences of reluctant speech. By definition, reluctant speech is responsive speech. This means that for the person to verbally respond, he or she must be asked for a verbal response. A low frequency of reluctant speech may reflect a low frequency of questions rather than a refusal to respond. This could be tested by increasing or decreasing the number of questions and observing the number of verbal replies. For example, if asked one question in each of five observation intervals and the client did not respond to any of the questions, this would indicate that the "low-Response count" was not related to the number of questions directed to the client. If the client responded to fewer than five questions, this would suggest that the number of verbal replies was related to factors other than an artificial ceiling imposed by the number of questions. An artificial ceiling, however, might be suspected if a client responded to each of the five questions. This could be tested by increasing the number of questions directed to the client in subsequent assessments. If the number of replies was observed to coincide with the number of questions, this would be evidence for a ceiling imposed by the questions.

Nonetheless, this observation could be interpreted as "positive" because the reluctant speech increased as the number of questions was increased. This would be additional evidence for the internal validity of the intervention – that reluctant speech occurred predictably to questions, even when the number of questions was increased. The process, as described above, is parallel to the changing criterion single subject research design (described in Tawney and Gast, 1984).

A scatter plot assessment, however, may not be useful for an intra-setting assessment of talking in the setting targeted for eliciting speech because of the zero occurrence of the speech acts. Ordinarily, there is no variation in speaking for time of day, people present, seat location and activity. A scatter plot assessment is useful, however, for targeting specific factors which are associated with the frequency of speaking in settings in which the client does speak.

Differences in the occurrence of responses might be observed in the setting targeted for eliciting speech, however, if covert responses were assessed. Self-observation and self-recording might be used to monitor covert responses such as "I wish I had spoken," or "I would speak if . . . ." This focus is useful in several ways:

• The self-monitoring and self-recording of statements of "intent" such as "I wanted to speak" make it possible to positively reinforce responses prior to the occurrence of speech acts which are directly observable by others. Otherwise internal statements of intent will go unrecognized and unreinforced. For example, statements of intent could be self-monitored and self-recorded and exchanged for backup reinforcers contingent on the client's accumulating a specified number of covert responses of intent.

- Self-monitored and self-recorded covert statements of intent to speak could readily be linked with specific environmental factors. This information is useful because the environmental factors coinciding with statements of intent can then be programmed into the target environment.
- Self-monitoring and self-recording of statements of intent may even contribute to the client's beginning to speak in the target environment through the reactive effects of self-observation.

CHAPTER 11

WHY-QUESTIONS: BEYOND DIRECT OBSERVATION

It is important to ask *when* rather than *if* people ask why-questions. Why-questions are a part of the search for causal understanding. If the experiences of people confirm their expectations, there is no need to ask about the "why" of an event or situation. For example, students with proven performance in artistic endeavours are expected to do well in artistic pursuits. With this expectation, success in artistic activities will probably not elicit why-questions.

FOCI OF WHY-QUESTIONS

Why-questions address (1) the locus of causality (whether the cause lies within the person or in the social context); (2) the controllability of the cause (whether the cause is subject to personal influence); and (3) causal stability (whether the cause will change or persist over time). The *frequency of why-questions* addressed by the client to each category gives information about the salience that the client places on each attribution category. If the clinician or researcher monitors the *serial position of the client's questions* a hypothesis may be generated about the priority that the client assigns to particular types of personal issues. Indeed, salience and priority data help the clinician to understand *how clients approach their problems*.

SURFACE AND CONTRASTING MEANINGS

Why-questions have a surface meaning as well as a contrasting meaning involving something else which could or should have happened. Temple (1988) argues that because of implied contrasts, why-questions may have several interpretations. For instance, the question "Why does Adam speak to his mother?" can be interpreted in several ways depending on what is taken as the relevant underlying question which is not directly asked. For example:
1. "Why does *Adam* speak to his mother?" [instead of someone else speaking to her];
2. "Why does Adam *speak* to his mother?" [instead of doing something else such as refusing to speak to her];

89

3. "Why does Adam speak to *his mother*?" [instead of speaking to someone else].

In many cases, however, one is simply puzzled about "why Adam speaks to his mother" without having in mind something else that could or should have happened.

THERAPEUTIC USE OF WHY-QUESTIONS

Wack (1977) cautions that when therapists ask why-questions, clients may perceive the "why" as the equivalent of "explain yourself" and respond as they would to a reprimand. Wack, therefore, suggests that a more productive approach is to substitute "how," "what," "where," and "how come" questions for "why" questions. According to Wack (1977), substitutes for why-questions include:

"How did you find yourself in that spot?", "What were you thinking/feeling when you did that?", "How often do you find yourself in that spot?", "When you do this how do you end up feeling?" (p.252).

The above excerpt illustrates the substitution option and shows how Wack's approach parallels the BASIC ID interview. For an explanation of the BASIC ID interview, the reader is referred to Chapter 12.

Hollender and Ford (1990) advise that "why" questions should be used sparingly. They claim that "what," or "when," or "how" questions serve the same purpose as why-questions in getting clients to elaborate on their problems. The position of Hollender and Ford (1990) is similar to the argument advanced by Wack (1977).

The therapist may ask why to obtain additional information, but patients may react as though their behavior is being criticized or their motives impugned. Accordingly, they may proceed to attempt to justify their actions. This problem in communication is so common that therapists should constantly be on the alert for it. If signs of it are detected, an immediate effort should be made to abort the misunderstanding by clarifying the matter. On occasion it may be possible and desirable to preclude such a misunderstanding by asking "Would you talk more about this subject?" instead of asking "Why?" (p. 72)

ADAPTIVE AND DEFENSIVE FUNCTIONS

Wong and Weiner (1981) review the adaptive and defensive functions of why-questions. They have this to say about the adaptive and defensive functions:

Perhaps defensive functioning predominates when one is publicly asked to give an explanation of a task already completed, whereas adaptive functioning prevails when there is a search for a solution to problems that may occur. In [the Wong and Weiner (1981) investigation], questions about internal and controllable causes (effort) for failure typically were followed by questions about possible coping actions. The adaptive advantage of this kind of bias in causal search is that one is motivated to plan constructive coping actions only when the cause is perceived as controllable by the actor (p. 658).

Clients can also ask why-questions. A question such as "if I only knew why I do not speak in class" often invites unproductive interchange. One solution in dealing with a why question is to ask the client to "change chairs, be your own therapist and answer the question" (Wack, 1977). The "change in chairs" technique (1) lets the therapist know if the question is genuine or if it is only part of self-defeating communication and (2) permits clients to use their skills in solving their problems. There is a potential danger in answering why-questions because the responses often are based on interpretation. The potential problems associated with interpretation are discussed under interpretation as translation and interpretation as process.

INTERPRETATION AS TRANSLATION

Freud believed that there were symbols in the unconscious which were uniform for all people. Unconscious symbols were seen as a primitive sort of inherited language. For Freud, "the unconscious consisted of thing-representations but when they were linked with words they could become conscious" (Saari, 1988, p. 379). Freud's notion of interpretation, then, involves the translation of meaning from one code to another – that is, from an unconscious code which does not involve words to one in which the symbol becomes conscious by being expressed in words. Interpretation is an event in which therapists assign meaning to the clients' verbal and nonverbal behavior and communicate the translations to them. The words "what you mean is" or "what I hear you saying is" indicate that the therapist is about to make a translation. If this model of interpretation is valid, one must account for how the therapist acquires the knowledge of the inherited symbolic code in order to translate the words of the client into the meaning embodied in the symbols. Piaget (cited in Saari, 1988), who disagreed with Freud about inherited unconscious symbols, believed that symbols were learned during the course of interaction with the environment.

INTERPRETATION AS CREATION OF MEANING

Therapeutic interpretation may also be viewed as a process of *helping clients to create meaning*. This position claims that interpretation is a process in which the client and the therapist negotiate meaning. This view of interpretation also holds that many *behavior problems involve deficits in the capacity to create meaning*. Numerous examples might be given to show that human beings will endure any "what" of living if they understand a "why." I remember attending an exciting lecture by Dr. Victor Frankel when I was an undergraduate student. He emphasized that to *suffer without meaning is intolerable*. Consistent with this position is the belief that the content of the meaning is secondary to the capacity to create meaning. Meaning is not inherent in a particular event or action. Meaning is constructed in the mind of the observer. According to Saari (1988) the process of *creating meaning* underlies therapy. The client and the therapist are involved in creating meaning and in *addressing or modifying the difficulties the client has in creating meaning*.

CHAPTER 12

ASSESSMENT OF ELECTIVELY MUTE BEHAVIOR

DELAY IN REFERRAL

The early investigation by Morris (1953) noted the delay between observing the mutistic behavior and referral for treatment. He asserted that this occurred because: (1) teachers may disregard milder forms of elective mutism and await spontaneous recovery and (2) electively mute children may be classified as mental defective because of the absence of a full investigation of the problem. According to Carr and Afnan (1989) the delay between the onset of elective mutism and referral for treatment is due to the family preferring to wait for the child to grow out of his or her mutism, and to use their own strategies to get the child to talk before seeking professional help.

INTERVIEWING ELECTIVELY MUTE PERSONS

Psychological literature does not address the interviewing of electively mute persons. The literature, however, does offer guidelines for interviewing mentally retarded persons which may be useful in interviewing silence users. Zero verbal responsiveness is a major problem associated with interviewing electively mute persons. If the person is electively mute, he or she should not be expected to respond to open-ended questions or to verbal multiple choice questions unless given the option of responding in writing to the open-ended questions, or pointing to the written or pictorial response options of multiple-choice questions. Figure 12.1 illustrates open-ended questions and two alternate techniques for questioning electively mute persons. Because the multiple choice format is highly successful in getting retarded persons to respond, it should be useful for interviewing people who elect not to speak.

Sigelman *et al.* (1982) compared open-ended questions with verbal and pictorial multiple choice questions. These authors reported that for mentally retarded persons the responsiveness was 100% to the pictorial multiple choice questions, 94.5% to the verbal multiple choice questions and 73.6% to the open-ended questions. Both types of multiple choice questions were superior to open-ended questions in getting mentally retarded persons to respond.

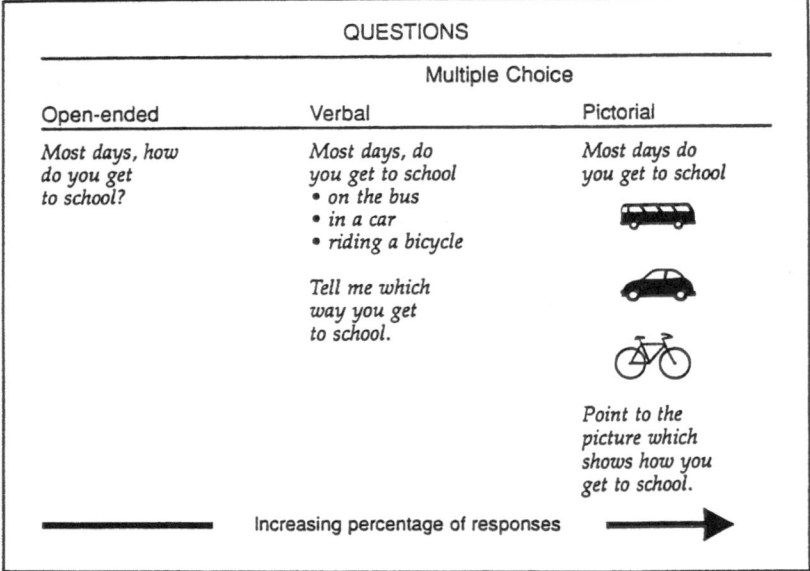

Fig. 12.1. Question format options.

Discussion

Another approach for interviewing electively mute children is an audio-tape consisting of a sequence of questions and "blank segments" to allow the client to record his or her answers. The sequence is similar to that used in an answering machine in which the message of the person called is followed by a space on the tape for the caller to leave a message.

As is illustrated in Fig. 12.2, the child listens to the questions at home and records his or her answer to each question on the blank segment of the audiotape which follows each question. This method of interviewing allows the client to answer the therapist's questions in a setting in which

Audiotape

| Question 1 | Blank segment to allow client's recording of answer | Question 2 | Blank segment to allow client's recording of answer |

Fig. 12.2. Question-space audio interview method.

he or she elects to speak. This procedure also provides an opportunity for positive self-modeling because, on playing back the recording, the client hears himself or herself speak in the presence of a person to whom he or she does not speak in face-to-face communication. I recognize, however, that the positive self-modeling is limited to the verbal component of the speech acts. An audiotape denies us access to the nonverbal behaviors of the speech-acts of the sender and receiver, and the physical setting of the communication. In order to enhance the effects of positive self-modeling, the child should be encouraged to listen to the audiotape in the presence of the clinician.

QUANTITATIVE MEASURES

Using a tape recorder permits the collection of four duration measures in addition to its use in biofeedback based interventions: (1) response duration measures for individual questions, (2) total speaking time during each session, (3) the latency or time between the end of the therapist's asking a question or prompts to make a sound and the beginning of the client's sound or verbal response and, as well, (4) the inter-response time between episodes of spontaneous speech. A word count or frequency measure could also be obtained from the audio recording. Successful treatment might be predicted to show a decrease in response latency, a decrease in inter-response time in spontaneous speech, an increase in the number and frequency of sounds or words spoken and an increase in the duration of verbal responses as treatment progressed.

There are a number of options for using a tape recorder. The child could take the tape recorder to the setting where he speaks and record samples of his spontaneous speech in this setting. This option would permit the therapist to compute latency and duration measures for spontaneous speech that occurred in a setting in which the client talks. The word count, latency and duration data from the setting in which the client talks would be useful baseline data to compare the child's verbal responses in non-speaking settings. Baseline data from settings in which the child talks would also be useful for setting realistic treatment goals in environments where you wish the client to speak. This data would enable interventions to be compared with: (1) a before treatment baseline obtained in the target environment and (2) a baseline obtained in a setting in which the client speaks.

The *content* of the tapes also provides useful information for designing interventions for elective mutism. Appelman *et al.* (1975) selected the words to use in the speech-language activities with their silent client based on the "words which the parents heard the child occasionally produce" (p. 6). These words could be used in a variety of ways – e.g., in word or sentence flash cards, in the mutual story-telling technique and in custom-designed excerpts for bibliotherapy sessions.

Direct Observation of Speaking Episodes of Electively Mute Persons

Joan Tough (1985) presents an unstructured diary, an elaborated diary and a check-list for appraising children's use of language. Diary-type jottings require the observer to identify the time of the child's speaking episodes, to record a brief description of the behavior and to summarize the observations for each day. The illustration of diary-type jottings in Table 12.1 combines behavioral descriptions with a concluding interpretative summary.

Table 12.1. Observations obtained by diary-type jottings.

Johnnie Smith	12th October 1975

9:05	Brought mother into classroom to see hamster. Shouted 'Can't I give him some apple Miss H.?" Ran after mother – waved. Joined Peter S. in sand – demanded sieve – some talk.
9:30	With Peter and Brian at slide. Shouting 'Watch me what I can do.' Each trying to outdo the other – friendly rivalry.
9:50	Sitting alone drinking milk; shows interest in blocks construction beside him. Pushes blocks over – shouts 'Sorry' as Bill threatens him.
10.:30	Absorbed in painting picture and has difficulty controlling brush. Speaks to Miss H. first. Replies 'It's my dad and that's his car.'
11:15	On outer edge of group listening to story. Restless, rolls on floor, Miss H. speaks to him, looks abashed and sucks his thumb.
11:40	Sees mother, leaves group, speaks to Miss H. 'Want my painting.' Runs to show it to mother.

Summary
Johnnie is rapidly adjusting to others. Quite confident with other children and teacher. Approaches and responds. Excitable and easily distracted. Needs help in listening with group. Must make a point of looking at books and telling story to him alone when possible.

Note: From *Listening to Children Talking* (p. 40) by J. Tough, 1985, London: Ward Lock Educational. Copyright 1985 by Ward Lock Educational. Reprinted with permission.

Discussion

The diary-type jottings method is useful if little is known about the client's electively mute behavior. The flexibility of the diary format is especially well suited for recording observations during expressive therapy. If the observer has obtained a pattern, he may find that the data enables him to use either the structured diary method or the checklist method. An admirable feature of the diary-type jottings is the separation of the observations from the summaries. This is important because if impressions rather than descriptions are initially recorded it is difficult, if not impossible, to make data-based interpretations. If it is useful to include tentative interpretations, the notation for indicating interpretations in specimen descriptions should be used.

Elaborated Diary Method

The structured diary method provides for the recording of the context of the behavior and the observed responses including utterances. Furthermore, the format "gives the [observer] some reminder of the points to be noted" (Tough, 1985, p. 40). But, in the sample entries, descriptions of behavior are combined with interpretations of behavior. I, therefore, recommend that the specimen description guidelines be used so that the functional

Table 12.2. Observations obtained by elaborated diary method.

Tom Reynolds: 14th October 1975

Time	Activity	Character of talk and behavior	Utterances heard
9:10	Mother pushes Tom into classroom – he stands alone, looking after her. I offer my hand and welcome him.	No speech: talks hand: comes to sand tray.	None
9:30	Still in sand: digging with hands, lets sand run through fingers.	Seems to be listening to Brian J. and Jimmie C.	None
10:10	Washing his hands slowly. No response when I speak to him.	Withdrawn – seems timid – watches other children.	None
11:00	Sitting in rocker alone. Miss B. asks Brian J. to rock with with.	Lowers head: looks apprehensively at Brian but rocks with him.	None
11:45	Stands looking out of window.	Tell him mother's coming soon: sucks his thumb.	

Summary
Tom was not seen to speak to anyone during the observations. Mother reports that he talks a lot at home. Some evidence that he is beginning to accept Brian J. Perhaps it would help if mother stayed longer. Will invite her to stay and help Tom to try out other activities.

Note: From *Listening to Children Talking* (p. 41) by J. Tough, 1985, London: Ward Lock Educational. Copyright 1985 by Ward Lock Educational. Reprinted with permission.

analysis can be applied to the entries. The system does not readily permit the determination of stimulus control, but it does provide a comprehensive picture of behavior which is ideally suited to observing electively mute individuals.

Discussion

I would like to caution that entries such as "talks easily" are not observations; rather they are interpretations of the observed behavior. It is difficult, if not impossible, to monitor progress by comparing interpretations. Therefore, comparisons should be made between behavioral descriptions if statements of progress are to be useful. An attractive feature of the elaborated diary method is that it is flexible enough to allow for recording the consequences of utterances. This means that hypotheses based on direct observations can be generated concerning the degree to which the response consequences increase, decrease or maintain the speech refusal.

Check-List Method

The third approach discussed by Tough (1985) is the check-list method. This approach to recording direct observations "takes the least time during actual observations, although more time must be spent on preparing the form" (Tough, 1985, p. 41). This approach also permits the practitioner to readily identify the occurrences and nonoccurrences of a variety of related responses. According to Tough (1985), practitioners who find the check-list method useful should not hesitate in deleting or adding items so that it suits their own particular situation (see Table 12.3).

MODELS OF BEHAVIOR ASSESSMENT

Introduction

There is a basic difference between traditional and behavioral assessment. When test responses are viewed as a sample of behavior, one assumes that they parallel the way in which a person is likely to behave in a non-test situation. Thus, if a person responds assertively on a test, one may assume that this or similar assertive behaviors occur in other situations. In a sample approach to assessment, the interest is in the behavior itself and in how it is affected by environmental conditions.

When test responses are viewed as signs, an inference is made that the performance is an indirect or symbolic manifestation of some other

Table 12.3. Observations obtained by check-list method.

Child's name: Wendy Brown   Date: 30th November 1975

Time of observation	9:30	10:00 5	10:3 5	11:0 0	11:1 5	12:10
Participation in classroom activity						
Child alone and not involved in any activity						
Child alone but watching others						
Child absorbed in some activity alone		x				
Child following own activity but aware of others						
Child participating in a group		x		x	x	x
Talk with others						
No talk observed						
Child playing and talking to self, not aware of others						
Child listening to others but not talking						
Child talking and aware of others but not requiring responses from them						
Child initiating conversation and seeking responses		x		x		
Child directing behavior of others		x				x
Child being directed by another						
Talk with adults						
Initiates conversation with teacher			x			
Responds when approached by teacher				x		
Maintains a dialogue easily				x		
Maintains a dialogue with difficulty						
Contributes when with teacher (in a group)				x		
General behavior characteristics						
Any particular features of behavior that emerge (e.g., friendly, confident, aggressive, dominant, shy, shows lack of concentration).	*Friendly, confident*					

Summary of observed behavior
Wendy appeared very confident and moved around the classroom easily, engaged in a variety of activities and completed each before moving on. She involved other children in conversation and responded eagerly with a lot of talk when the teacher approached her.

Note: From *Listening to Children Talking* (p. 42) by J. Tough, 1985, London: Ward Lock Educational. Copyright 1985 by Ward Lock Educational. Reprinted with permission.

characteristic. An example is black clouds and a heavy downpour of rain together with the noticeable absence of rainwear, umbrella and a visible refuge, such as a doorway, in the projective drawing of a person in the rain. According to the guidelines for interpreting the drawings, the black clouds and the heavy rainfall are signs of stress while the absence of protection against the rain indicates minimal strategies for coping with stress. In summary, behavioral characteristics are inferred from the test responses. The sign approach asks about motives and characteristics that act together to produce the observed behavior whereas the sample approach asks about environmental variables that influence the frequency, intensity and duration of behavior.

Kanfer and Saslow Model

There are several behavioral assessment models. One such approach is that of Kanfer and Saslow (1969). Morganstern and Telvin (1981) have provided an excellent overview of Kanfer and Saslow's assessment method. I have, therefore, included it here as a prelude to my discussion of the application of their method to the behavioral assessment of elective mutism:

In probably the most extensive assessment scheme, Kanfer and Saslow (1969) described an approach that incorporated variables from both the client's current situation and past history. They emphasized, however, that historical information is relevant only to the extent that it facilitates the description of current problematic behaviors and future therapeutic interventions. In order to accomplish this task, Kanfer and Saslow suggested an examination of each of the following areas: (1) analysis of the problem situation (including behavioral excesses, deficits, and assets); (2) clarification of the problem situation that maintains the targeted behaviors; (3) a motivational analysis; (4) a developmental analysis (including biological, sociological, and behavioral spheres); (5) a self-control analysis; (6) an analysis of social relationships; and (7) an analysis of the social-cultural-physical environment. A noteworthy contribution of Kanfer and Saslow's outline is the inclusion of an assessment of the client's strengths, assets, skills, and talents (p. 74).

Kanfer and Saslow's model initially focuses on determining client strengths. The second major focus is determining if the problem is a behavioral excess or a behavioral deficit. Responses which occur with too great a frequency, for too long a duration, or at an intensity which is uncomfortable for the patient or others are termed behavioral excesses (Kanfer and Saslow, 1969). Silences of long duration are an example of a behavioral excess for the problem of elective mutism. The second component of Kanfer and Saslow's approach is problem clarification. For elective mutism this part of the behavioral assessment revolves around determining the consequences of the silence-user role for the patient and for people in the life of the patient.

The third area of the model is motivational analysis. The initial focus is on obtaining information about events that are positively reinforcing for the patient (Kanfer and Saslow, 1969). In the case of elective mutism, the client is asked to estimate the frequency or the amount of time that he or she uses silence. A reinforcement menu based on potential reinforcers for electively mute behavior is helpful if the client is unable to identify positively reinforcing stimuli. Second, motivational analysis is also aimed at providing information about events that the patient seeks to escape or avoid. Third, data is obtained about how patients account for their electively mute behavior. In other words, the focus is on determining how patients account for the inappropriate use of silence.

The fourth focus is developmental analysis. First, significant biological events such as previous or present illnesses, and low energy which might interfere with the goals of intervention are assessed. Second, assessment is aimed at determining if the patient's behavior, attitudes or beliefs are congruent with family and community norms. Potential role conflicts are also investigated. For example, problems associated with attending school and not talking at school are delineated. Third, additional questions include: (1) Has the patient's behavior recently changed?, (2) If so, how?, and (3) Are these behaviors linked to specific events in the family or at school? (Kanfer and Saslow, 1969).

The fifth area deals with analysis of self-control. The purpose of this guideline is to assess how the patient attempts to control his or her problematic behavior (Kanfer and Saslow, 1969). Sample questions might include: What do you think you could do to get yourself to speak when you are afraid of being negatively criticized? Or, what could you do to express your anger directly rather than using prolonged silences to express anger? In addition, the therapist determines if the client typically exercises positive control (e.g., "rewarding" herself by positive self-statements) or aversive control (e.g., not talking because of "possible" negative consequences).

The focus of the sixth area of assessment is social relationships. Kanfer and Saslow delineate five items within this category:

- Who are the most significant people in the patient's current environment? To which persons or groups is he most responsive? Who facilitates constructive behaviors? Who provokes antagonistic or problematic behaviors? Can these relationships be categorized according to dimensions which clarify the patient's behavioral patterns (e.g., does a patient respond in a submissive or hostile way to all older men)?
- In these relationships, by use of what reinforcers do the participants influence each other? For example, analysis may reveal a father who always bails out a delinquent son whose public punishment would be embarrassing to the father. Is the cessation of positive reinforcement or onset of punishment clearly signaled?
- What does the patient expect of these people in words and in action? On what does he base his verbal expectations?

- What do these people expect of the patient? Is there consistency between the patient's and others' expectations for him?
- How can these people who can influence the patient participate in treatment? (p. 436)

The final focus relates the assessment of the influence of the physical, social and cultural environment. The question, "What are the norms in the patient's social milieu for behaviors about which there is a complaint?" (p. 436) is important for elective mutism. The excessive use of silence in the school setting, for example, violates the "participation rule." Indeed, the child's failure to be guided by this rule may be one of the reasons for his or her referral to health professionals. The Kanfer and Saslow (1969) procedure queries the consistency or lack of consistency of the norms for specific behaviors in the various settings of the patient (Kanfer and Saslow, 1969). Here we are concerned with the excessive use of silences which are encouraged in one setting but not in another.

Lazarus' BASIC ID

Lazarus' technique of behavior assessment focuses on seven different interrelated areas. In the BASIC ID assessment: B = behavior, A = affect, S = sensations, I = imagery, C = cognitions, I = interpersonal relationships, D = drugs.

In the behavior component, verbal or motoric responses are examined and the antecedents and consequences of identified responses are obtained through direct observation or self-report (Lazarus, 1976). Relevant questions include: (1) What are the events that provoke the silence user role? and (2) What are the consequences of the elective mutism for the silence user and the silence receiver? The affect dimension deals with the identification of events that elicit fear, anger, sadness and other emotions to provide a profile of situations associated with positive as well as negative feelings. It is also important to determine what causes a patient to apply a specific label to a particular experience or event. The clinician should be aware of potential interrelationships among the assessment components. For example, the interrelationship between behavior and affect could be determined by asking: "How do you feel when you are asked a question and you do not reply?"

The third component deals with sensation. Sensations refer to physiological experiences such as nausea, pain, headaches and dizziness. In addition, questions may be asked about appetite, energy level, and sleep. The fourth component is imagery. By imagery, Lazarus means the "mental pictures" that the client reports which influence his life. The accurate assessment of imagery and sensation depends on clearly distinguishing between the two. Imagery primarily refers to mental pictures of events while sensation refers to particular physiological responses to real or imagined events. For example, a patient imagines herself speaking to a stranger (imagery component) while simultaneously reporting an upset stomach (sensation component). In the case of a child, it is important for the therapist to determine if the child can distinguish between real and imaginary events. Lazarus frequently involves the patient in various imagery exercises. The therapist might instruct the patient to "picture yourself in your classroom at school." In addition, the client might be asked to focus on the feelings associated with not talking when the teacher asks a question.

The fifth area of assessment is cognition. In this component, the therapist obtains information about the patient's thinking. This information comes from self-report as does the data for the other components. The therapist especially attempts to identify irrational thinking and internalized self-defeating sentences. In addition, the therapist attempts to pinpoint personal and family "rules" (Lazarus, 1976). Rules that play a dominant role in the life of the patient can be readily identified by statements that include the word "should." For example, the statement "I should be quiet when I am with people older than myself" suggests that the patient's early socialization included the guideline that "Children should be seen and not heard." A number of these "should" rules are unadaptive and contribute to elective mutism. Examples include "I *should* only answer a question if I am sure I am right" and "Everyone *should* agree with what I say." The cognitive component also focuses on how the clients attempt to explain their behavior. For example, students who are fearful of speaking in class may indicate that they do not speak because they are not "smart" enough. This statement is vague and, therefore, the clients should be asked to explain what they mean by "smart." For example "Do you want to tell me what you would have to be like to be "smart?"[1]

A number of other issues which can be dealt with in the cognitive component include religious beliefs, and locus of control. Locus of control can be visualized on a continuum marked by externality at one end and by internality at the other end. Because of the implications for intervention planning, it is important to determine the predominant locus of control used by the client. Clients with an external locus of control believe that events have minimal connection to their personal effort or behavior. Clients who have an internal locus of control believe that what happens to them is dependent on what they do.

The sixth component covers interpersonal relationships. Elective mutism especially applies to this component of the BASIC ID assessment. It is advisable to obtain information not only through self-report but also through direct observation of the client in interpersonal situations. Verbal and non-verbal behavior is examined not only for content but also for other features which might interfere with effective communication. For example, the patient's vocalizations such as verbal segregates ("uh," "um," "uh-huh") and vocal characteristics such as repeatedly clearing the throat may elicit visible annoyance from other persons. The seventh section is designated by the word drugs. The "D" component of the BASIC ID refers to much more than substance abuse. The "D" aspect includes physical appearance including dress, speech disorders, psychomotor skill and information about exercise, sleep and nutrition.

I do not recommend that the therapist employ only one model of behavior assessment; rather, a comprehensive assessment may involve several approaches. I prefer, however, Lazarus' BASIC ID model because of its multi-dimensional focus on the experience of the person. Indeed, the responses on the various dimensions of the BASIC ID constitute a useful way of assessing the experience of the silence user.

NOTE

[1] The question is posed as a conversational postulate (polite command). In their two-volume work, *The Structure of Magic*, Bandler and Grinder provide guidelines which can be readily applied to behavioral interviewing. In addition, their discussion of representational systems is particularly helpful. What sensory modality does the patient use in representing her experience? For example, one patient uses the visual modality ("Do you *see* what I mean?") to ask "Do you understand me?" while another patient uses the auditory modality ("Do you hear what I am saying?") to ask the same question. Knowing a patient's most used representational system is useful in establishing effective communication. As practitioners, if we can be sensitive to the representational systems of the patient, we then have the choice of translating our communication into her system.

CHAPTER 13

ELECTIVE MUTISM INTERVIEW SCHEDULE

CONTENT VALIDITY

The semi-structured interview format should encourage the interviewer to probe the response options endorsed by the informants. The items are based on a review of the literature and the source, on which each question is based, is indicated. Sampling of the relevant features of elective mutism ensures that the questions have content validity. The emphasis on content validity is consistent with the sample approach to assessment in behavior analysis.

GUIDELINES

The questions for a behavioral assessment of elective mutism are intended for speech-language pathologists, psychiatrists, psychologists, social workers and guidance counsellors. The schedule can be used as a guide for interviewing significant persons in the life of the electively mute person. These questions with minor rewording can be asked the silence user by a person with whom the electively mute person typically speaks. If the interview schedule is administered by a person other than a therapist, it is essential that this individual be given training.

There are several advantages to having an individual that the electively mute person knows administer the interview schedule. First, since rapport is already established, this would not be an issue. Second, a person who has direct contact with the silence user is in a good position to comment or elaborate on the client's responses. Third, since caretakers are frequently asked to cooperate in therapy it is advisable to involve them in the assessment phase of treatment.

For several questions, one of the response options is "don't know" (DK). Questions answered by DK are useful in several ways. First, it alerts the interviewer to the fact that the respondent may be attempting to conceal information. Second, the DK option also has the advantage of permitting informants to conceal information without subjecting them to embarrassment. Third, it suggests to the interviewer that an informant may have had insufficient opportunity to observe the client and is, therefore, unable to provide an answer other than DK. In the case of insufficient observation, the interviewer should instruct the informant to monitor the client's behavior.

A number of the questions have response options which are "labels for behavior" such as "If yes, what did the teacher say or do to get him/her to talk at school?" Five options are provided – encourage him/her, become angry with him/her, threaten him/her, punish him/her and change his/her classroom. For each option, it is important to identify exactly what the person did. For example, querying the punishment option might reveal that when the client refused to answer, the teacher had him sit in a chair facing the wall.

DIRECTIONS

Above each of the three columns of boxes, the interviewer is required to indicate the identity of the informant or the identity of the intervention phase. The three boxes before each question can be used in two ways: First, this format enables the therapist to obtain information from three different informants and to conveniently record it so that comparisons and contrasts among the informants' responses can be determined. Second, the boxes beside each question can also be used to conveniently record the process and outcome of therapy. Responses to selected questions before, during, and at the conclusion of therapy may be useful dependent variable measures to assess the effectiveness of the intervention. Or alternately, one of the columns could be used to obtain follow-up data to determine the long-term effects of the intervention.

CHARTING DEPENDENT VARIABLE MEASURES

Clinicians may wish to use an approach which is based on observation but which does not involve counting the number of words spoken or timing the duration of speaking episodes. With minor modifications a number of questions can be made into rating items. Descriptors such as "not true as far as I know," "somewhat, or sometimes true," and "very true or often true" could be substituted for response options which are indicated for specific questions on the interview schedule. Numerical values such as 0, 1 and 2 could also be assigned to each of the above descriptions which would permit quantification and charting of the responses.

An innovative use of the inventory, for example, would be to have the client assess himself or herself on selected items, such as eye contact, during the various phases of treatment. The therapist could then plot the client's self-report data on the same graph as the therapist's ratings. If there are major discrepancies between the therapist ratings and the client self-ratings, the therapist can explore the plausible reasons for the discrepancies.

The discussion here is exemplary rather than inclusive. Client and/or

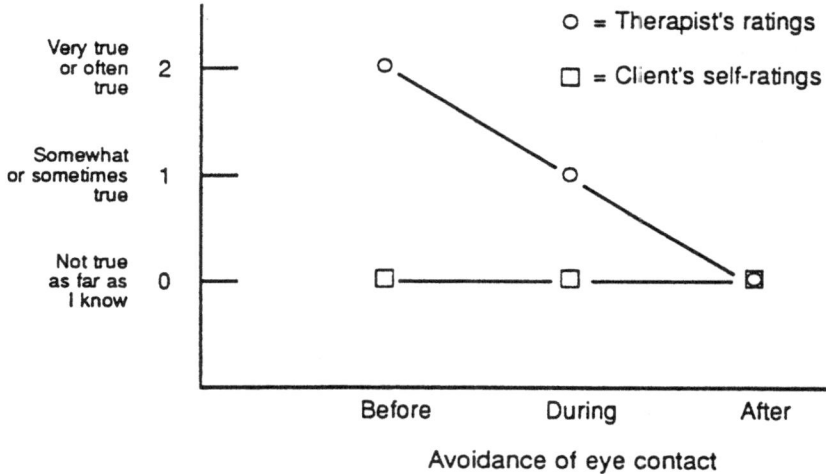

Fig. 13.1. Client self-assessment and therapist assessment of client on item based on interview schedule.

therapist ratings from other questions could be similarly used as dependent variables.

Responses to specific questions associated with the characteristics of the elective mutism in a particular client can be used as dependent variables to monitor intervention effects. For example, suppose that the before treatment rating on a particular item such as avoidance of eye contact was

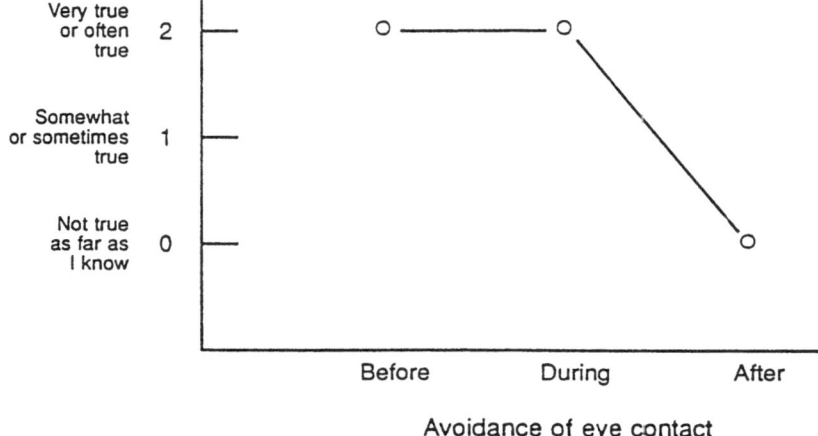

Fig. 13.2. Example of using a specific item from interview schedule as dependent variable to monitor intervention effects.

"very true or often true." Using a numerical system where 0 = not true as far as I know, 1 = somewhat or sometimes true and 2 = very true or often true, it would be possible to chart the client's performance before, during and at the conclusion of treatment. Figure 13.2 shows how a specific item from the interview guide can be used as a dependent variable to monitor client progress.

1. SILENCE ONSET

The first section of the interview schedule is intended to explore the characteristics associated with the onset of the client's elective mutism. The attributions of the client and other people concerning the purpose of the mutistic response is also a target for assessment.

1-1. How old was _____ when you first noticed his/her electively mute behavior? [Wergeland, 1979; Wright et al., 1985. Wright, 1968]	☐ ☐ ☐	Don't know
	☐ ☐ ☐	2–3 years
	☐ ☐ ☐	4–5 years
	☐ ☐ ☐	6–7 years
	☐ ☐ ☐	8–9 years
	☐ ☐ ☐	Other (specify)
1-2. Has _____ ever said why he/she does not talk in/at _____ ? [Ambrosino & Alessi, 1979; Bednar, 1974; Colligan et al., 1977; Goll, 1979; Kaplan & Escoll, 1973; Wilkins, 1985; Wright, 1968]	☐ ☐ ☐	No
	☐ ☐ ☐	Yes (specify)

1-3. Do you believe there has been any event that may have led to the onset of the mutism?
[Barlow et al., 1984; Kolvin & Fundudis, 1981; Wergeland, 1979; Wright et al., 1985; Wright, 1968]

☐ ☐ ☐ Hospitalization

☐ ☐ ☐ Separation/Divorce

☐ ☐ ☐ Death of family member

☐ ☐ ☐ Birth of sibling

☐ ☐ ☐ Accident or injury (specify)

☐ ☐ ☐ Other (specify)

1-4. Can you identify the last time he/she spoke in school?
[Brown & Doll, 1988]

☐ ☐ ☐ Yes

☐ ☐ ☐ No

☐ ☐ ☐ Don't know

☐ ☐ ☐ Other (specify)

1-5. If "yes" I wonder if you can tell me about the last time he/she spoke in your class?

☐ ☐ ☐

1-6. Has _____ offered a reason   ☐ ☐ ☐   No
      for not talking in _____ ?
      [Ambrosino & Alessi, 1979;
      Bednar, 1974; Colligan et al.,   ☐ ☐ ☐   Yes (specify)
      1977; Goll, 1979, Kaplan
      & Escoll, 1973; Wilkins,
      1985; Wright, 1968]

1-7. In your opinion what purpose   ☐ ☐ ☐   Attention-getting (explain)
      does the silence have for
      _____ ?
      [Reed, 1963]   ☐ ☐ ☐   Anxiety-reducing (explain)

                                         ☐ ☐ ☐   Self-controlling (explain)

                                         ☐ ☐ ☐   Expression of anger or
                                                    disagreement (explain)

                                         ☐ ☐ ☐   Other (specify)

                                         ☐ ☐ ☐   Don't know

2. PLAY AND SOCIAL BEHAVIOR

The questions in this section allow the clinician to explore the child's interactions during play. The items are intended to identify the typical pattern(s) in the play and social behavior of the child. These observations, in turn, may be compared and contrasted with the behavior of the other children from the same setting.

2-1. Have you ever observed _____ □ □ □   Yes
       playing with other children?
       [Pustrom & Speers, 1964;
       Wergeland, 1979]   □ □ □   No

2-2. If yes, in your estimation   □ □ □   Everyday
       how often does _____
       play with other children   □ □ □   4–6 times per week
       during the course of
       a week?   □ □ □   2–3 times per week

                                       □ □ □   once per week

                                       □ □ □   rarely (explain)

NOTES:

☐ ☐ ☐	☐ ☐ ☐	☐ ☐ ☐

2-3. Does _____ speak to
his/her peers during play?
[Brown & Doll, 1988]

☐ ☐ ☐ Yes

☐ ☐ ☐ No

☐ ☐ ☐ Don't know

☐ ☐ ☐ Other (specify)

2-4. If "no," has _____ ever
told you why she/he does
not talk to his peers
during play?

☐ ☐ ☐ Yes

☐ ☐ ☐ No

2-5. If "yes," I wonder if you
can tell me about what
_____ said about this?

☐ ☐ ☐

2-6. Do you have an opinion
about why _____ does
not talk to other students
during play at school?

☐ ☐ ☐ No

☐ ☐ ☐ Yes

☐ ☐ ☐ Don't know

☐ ☐ ☐ Other (specify)

2-7. If "yes," in your opinion
      why does _____ not talk
      to the other students during
      play at school?

NOTES:

3. REFERRAL OF THE SILENCE USER

This section of the interview schedule explores the reason(s) for referring the person for professional help. Questions relate to the period of language acquisition, the psychosocial characteristics of the setting in which the person elects to be silent and the reactions of people to the person's speech refusal. Several items address the attempts by teachers and parents to elicit speech.

	☐ ☐ ☐		

3-1.	With reference to _____ voluntary mutism, has he/she ever received treatment from another professional? [Colligan et al., 1977; Pustrom & Speers, 1964; Wergeland, 1979]	☐ ☐ ☐ ☐ ☐ ☐	Yes (specify) No
3-2.	What made you refer _____ for treatment?	☐ ☐ ☐	

NOTES:

3-3. How would you describe
      _____ language
      development?
      [Goll, 1979; Parker et al.,
      1960; Wilkins, 1985]

☐ ☐ ☐   Normal

☐ ☐ ☐   Delayed

☐ ☐ ☐   Articulation problems

☐ ☐ ☐   Stuttering

☐ ☐ ☐   Other (specify)

3-4. Did _____ need to be
      encouraged to speak
      when he/she first started
      talking?

☐ ☐ ☐   Yes (explain)

☐ ☐ ☐   No (explain)

☐ ☐ ☐   Don't know

3-5. Would you like to tell me
      where _____ elects to
      be silent?

☐ ☐ ☐   In class

☐ ☐ ☐   On the playground

☐ ☐ ☐   On the way to school

☐ ☐ ☐   On the way from school

☐ ☐ ☐   At home

☐ ☐ ☐   Other (specify)

☐ ☐ ☐

3-6. Has_____ teachers ever   ☐ ☐ ☐   Yes (explain)
      expressed concern to you
      about his/her mutism?
                                          ☐ ☐ ☐   No (explain)

3-7. If "yes," what did the   ☐ ☐ ☐   Encourages him/her (explain)
      teacher say or do to get
      _____ to speak?
      [Colligan et al., 1977;   ☐ ☐ ☐   Threaten him/her (explain)
      Nolan & Pence, 1970;
      Pustrom & Speers, 1964;
      Ruzicka & Sackin, 1974;   ☐ ☐ ☐   Punish him/her (explain)
      Barlow et al., 1984]

                                          ☐ ☐ ☐   Use Token reinforcement
                                                   (explain)

                                          ☐ ☐ ☐   Use time-out with him/her
                                                   (explain)

                                          ☐ ☐ ☐   Predicts he/she will
                                                   "outgrow" the problem
                                                   (explain)

                                          ☐ ☐ ☐   Other (specify)

3-8. What was your reaction   ☐ ☐ ☐   Surprise (explain)
      when you discovered that
      _____ does not
      speak in _____ ?   ☐ ☐ ☐   Not surprised (explain)

                                      ☐ ☐ ☐   Anger
                                      ☐ ☐ ☐   Fear
                                      ☐ ☐ ☐   Disappointment
                                      ☐ ☐ ☐   Other

3-9. Have you or a family   ☐ ☐ ☐   Yes
      member tried to get
      _____ to speak
      in _____?   ☐ ☐ ☐   No

NOTES:

4. FAMILY AND THE COMMUNITY

This component of the interview schedule addresses the nature and the extent of the family's communication outside the family and home. The way in which the client responds to strangers is also a target for assessment.

	▯ ▯ ▯	
4-1.	Do you have friends whom you see on a regular basis? [Meyers, 1984]	☐ ☐ ☐ Yes ☐ ☐ ☐ No
4-2.	Would you like to identify the people that you see on a regular basis?	☐ ☐ ☐ Relatives ☐ ☐ ☐ Friends ☐ ☐ ☐ Other (specify)

NOTES:

4-3. Check the following statements which describe the verbal behavior of _____ in the presence of visitors to your home.

☐ ☐ ☐ Greets relatives

☐ ☐ ☐ Greets friends

☐ ☐ ☐ Greets strangers

☐ ☐ ☐ Answers questions directed to him/her by relatives

☐ ☐ ☐ Answers questions directed to him/her by friends

☐ ☐ ☐ Answers questions directed to him/her by strangers

☐ ☐ ☐ Initiates conversation with relatives

☐ ☐ ☐ Initiates conversation with friends

☐ ☐ ☐ Initiates conversation with strangers

NOTES:

	▢▢▢	

4-4. What does _____ typically   ▢ ▢ ▢   Hides
      do when a stranger visits the
      home?   ▢ ▢ ▢   Leaves the room

                                     ▢ ▢ ▢   Cries

                                     ▢ ▢ ▢   Seeks comfort of mother

                                     ▢ ▢ ▢   Seeks comfort of father

                                     ▢ ▢ ▢   Other (specify)

4-5. Is there anyone in _____   ▢ ▢ ▢   No
      immediate family who could
      be described as quiet to the   ▢ ▢ ▢   Yes (specify)
      point where he/she rarely
      speaks?
      [Goll, 1979; Meyers, 1984]
                                     ▢ ▢ ▢   Uncertain (explain)

4-6. Does _____ take part in any ▢ ▢ ▢   Yes (specify)
      activities outside the home?
      [Meyers, 1984]
                                     ▢ ▢ ▢   No (explain)

4-7. How long has _____
lived at his/her current
address?

☐ ☐ ☐ 10 or more years

☐ ☐ ☐ 6–9 years

☐ ☐ ☐ 4–5 years

☐ ☐ ☐ 2–3 years

☐ ☐ ☐ 1 year

☐ ☐ ☐ less than a year

4-8. Is a language other than
English spoken in _____
home?
[Bednar, 1974; Calhoun
& Koenig, 1973; Conrad
et al., 1974]

☐ ☐ ☐ Yes (specify)

☐ ☐ ☐ No

NOTES:

5. COMMUNICATION OF THE SILENCE USER WITHIN THE FAMILY

Questions are directed at the form and frequency of communication within the family. The purpose is to provide an estimate of reluctant speech, self-initiated speech, low volume speech (whispering), and the frequency of normal speech acts within the family. Information is solicited either directly or through an informant to identify, if and how, the setting and the behavior of others needs to change in order for the client to talk. In addition to obtaining answers to the questions, it is desirable to obtain audio recordings of the child's verbal communication from settings in which he or she talks to permit the formulation of realistic treatment goals.

5-1. Does _____ talk at home? [Nolan & Pence, 1970; Wergeland, 1979]	☐ ☐ ☐ Yes
	☐ ☐ ☐ No
	☐ ☐ ☐ Rarely (explain)

NOTES:

5-2. How would you describe _____ behavior at home?
[Nolan & Pence, 1970; Reed, 1963; Wright, 1968]

☐ ☐ ☐ Obedient/Co-operative (describe)

☐ ☐ ☐ Defiant (describe)

☐ ☐ ☐ Withdrawn (describe)

☐ ☐ ☐ Passive-Aggressive (describe)

☐ ☐ ☐ Other (specify)

5-3. To whom does _____ speak?
[Reed, 1963]

☐ ☐ ☐ Mother

☐ ☐ ☐ Father

☐ ☐ ☐ Sister(s)

☐ ☐ ☐ Brother(s)

☐ ☐ ☐ Non-family (specify)

5-4. How would you describe _____ talking at home?

☐ ☐ ☐   Echolalic speech

☐ ☐ ☐   Reluctant speech

☐ ☐ ☐   Self-initiated speech

☐ ☐ ☐   Electively mute

☐ ☐ ☐   Whispers (low volume speech)

5-5. Does _____ verbally protest when another person calls him/her names?

☐ ☐ ☐   Yes

☐ ☐ ☐   No

☐ ☐ ☐   Don't know

5-6. Does _____ verbally protest when another person takes something which belongs to him/her?

☐ ☐ ☐   Yes

☐ ☐ ☐   No

☐ ☐ ☐   Don't know

NOTES:

5-7. Does ————— verbally
protest when another
person strikes him/her?

☐ ☐ ☐   Yes

☐ ☐ ☐   No

☐ ☐ ☐   Don't know

☐ ☐ ☐   Other occasions (specify)

5-8. Have you attempted to
get ————— to talk
in the target setting?

☐ ☐ ☐   Yes

☐ ☐ ☐   No

NOTES:

<table>
<tr><td></td><td colspan="3">☐ ☐ ☐</td><td></td></tr>
</table>

5-9.	If "yes," what have you done to get _____ to talk outside of the home? [Nolan & Pence, 1970; Rosenberg & Lindblad, 1978; Wergeland, 1979; Williamson et al., 1977]	☐ ☐ ☐ Encourage him/her (explain) ☐ ☐ ☐ Become angry with him/her (explain) ☐ ☐ ☐ Threaten him/her (explain) ☐ ☐ ☐ Punish him/her (explain) ☐ ☐ ☐ Other (specify)
5-10.	Did _____ ever say what would have to happen for him/her to begin to speak in the target setting?	☐ ☐ ☐ Yes ☐ ☐ ☐ No
5-11.	If "yes," what did _____ say would have to happen for him/her to talk?	☐ ☐ ☐

6. TELEPHONE USE OF THE SILENCE USER

The aim of this section of the interview guide is to determine if the client will talk to someone whom he can hear but cannot see. The data has implications for selecting a telephone for play therapy, for positive self-modeling and for interventions based on gradually exposing the person to the settings in which he or she is silent.

6-1.	If asked to answer the telephone with whom will he/she speak?	☐ ☐ ☐	Mother
		☐ ☐ ☐	Father
		☐ ☐ ☐	Grandmother
		☐ ☐ ☐	Grandfather
		☐ ☐ ☐	Aunt
		☐ ☐ ☐	Uncle
		☐ ☐ ☐	Sibling
		☐ ☐ ☐	Cousin
		☐ ☐ ☐	Close Friend
		☐ ☐ ☐	Other (specify)

NOTES:

6-2. Will _____ answer the telephone?
[Parker et al., 1960; Rosenberg & Lindblad, 1978; Williamson et al., 1977]

☐ ☐ ☐ Yes

☐ ☐ ☐ No

☐ ☐ ☐ Sometimes (explain)

6-3. Will _____ make a telephone call on his/her own?

☐ ☐ ☐ Yes

☐ ☐ ☐ No

☐ ☐ ☐ Rarely (specify)

6-4. If "yes," who does he/she call?

☐ ☐ ☐ Family member (specify)

☐ ☐ ☐ Non-family member (specify)

NOTES:

7. COMMUNICATION OF THE SILENCE USER IN THE TARGET SETTING

This section of the interview focuses on the gestural communication and the speech-acts of the client in the setting in which he or she elects to be silent. In addition to obtaining answers to the questions, it is useful to record samples of the verbal behavior of several other students in a variety of learning and social activities. This permits the clinician to make comparisons between the client's pattern of communication and the communication pattern of children from the same setting.

7-1. Does _____ speak to his/her peers? [Brown & Doll, 1988]

☐ ☐ ☐ Yes

☐ ☐ ☐ No

☐ ☐ ☐ Don't know

☐ ☐ ☐ Other (specify)

NOTES:

7-2. If "no," has _____ ever   ☐ ☐ ☐   Yes
      indicated why he/she does
      not talk to his/her peers?   ☐ ☐ ☐   No

                                           If "yes," I wonder if you can tell me
                                           about what he/she said about this?

                                           If "no," why do you think he/she
                                           does not talk to his/her peers?

7-3. How does _____ indicate   ☐ ☐ ☐   Whispers
      that he/she wants something
      when in a setting in which   ☐ ☐ ☐   Gestures
      he/she does not speak?
      [Colligan et al., 1977;   ☐ ☐ ☐   Writes
      Parker et al., 1960]
                                          ☐ ☐ ☐   Vocalizations – not words
                                                    (e.g., sounds such as cough-
                                                    ing, throat clearing, etc.)

                                          ☐ ☐ ☐   Helps himself /herself
                                                    independent of others

                                          ☐ ☐ ☐   Other (specify)

NOTES:

7-4. Can you identify the last time _____ spoke in school?
[Brown & Doll, 1988]

☐ ☐ ☐   Yes

☐ ☐ ☐   No

☐ ☐ ☐   Don't know

☐ ☐ ☐   Other (specify)

7-5. If "yes," I wonder if you can tell me about the last time he/she spoke in your class.

☐ ☐ ☐

7-6. Does _____ respond with gestures if instructed to do so? (e.g., nod his/her head for "Yes" – move his/her head from side-to-side for "no.")
[Brown & Doll, 1988]

☐ ☐ ☐   Yes

☐ ☐ ☐   No

☐ ☐ ☐   Don't know

☐ ☐ ☐   Other (explain)

7-7. If "yes," can you identify the gestures which he/she typically uses?

☐ ☐ ☐

7-8. Does _____ exhibit eye contact when you are talking to him/her?

☐ ☐ ☐   Yes

☐ ☐ ☐   No

☐ ☐ ☐   Don't know

8. REACTIONS OF PEERS TO THE SILENCE USER

This part of the interview schedule permits the clinician to record the reactions of other people to the client's use of silence.

	□□ □
8-1. How do other people react to _____ silence? [Bauermeister & Jemail, 1975; Pustrom & Speers, 1964; Ruzicka & Sackin, 1974]	□ □ □ Helpful (explain)
	□ □ □ Unfriendly (explain)
	□ □ □ Ignore (explain)
	□ □ □ Other (specify)

NOTES:

9. INFORMAL TREATMENTS

It is important for clinicians to determine if informal remediations have been applied in the past. If they have been applied, it is important to obtain a detailed account of the informal interventions. The impressions of the informants about the informal treatments to which the client has been exposed will be useful in designing alternative treatments.

9-1. Have you tried to get
_____ to talk in the
target setting?

☐ ☐ ☐ Yes

☐ ☐ ☐ No

☐ ☐ ☐ Other (specify)

NOTES:

9-2. If "yes," what have you   ☐ ☐ ☐   Encourage him/her (specify)
      done to get _____ to
      talk in the target setting?
      [Nolan & Pence, 1970;   ☐ ☐ ☐   Threaten him/her (specify)
      Rosenberg & Lindblad,
      1978; Wergeland, 1979;
      Williamson, et al., 1977]

                                       ☐ ☐ ☐   Punish him/her (specify)

                                       ☐ ☐ ☐   Become angry with him/her
                                                 (specify)

                                       ☐ ☐ ☐   Other (specify)

NOTES:

9-3. What does the teacher say
      or do to get _____ to
      talk at school?
      [Colligan et al., 1977;
      Nolan & Pence, 1970;
      Pustrom & speers, 1964;
      Ruzicka & Sackin, 1974;
      and Kehle et al., 1990]

☐ ☐ ☐ Encourages him/her (specify)

☐ ☐ ☐ Change of classroom
        (specify)

☐ ☐ ☐ Theatens him/her (specify)

☐ ☐ ☐ Punishes him/her (specify)

☐ ☐ ☐ Becomes angry with him/her
        (specify)

☐ ☐ ☐ Other (specify)

10. TREATMENT BY QUALIFIED PROFESSIONALS

This section is designed to permit the therapist to obtain information from family members about the nature and characteristics of the previous treatments and the status of the client at the conclusion of previous treatment(s). The data will assist the clinician in avoiding the pitfalls of the previous treatment(s) and in designing a treatment for the client which has a greater likelihood of being effective.

10-1.   Has_____ received
        professional help for   ☐ ☐ ☐   Yes
        his/her speech-refusal?
                                       ☐ ☐ ☐   No

                                       ☐ ☐ ☐   Don't know

NOTES:

10-2.	If "yes," tell me about the treatment. [Norman & Broman, 1970; Nolan & Pence, 1970; Brown & Doll, 1988]	☐ ☐ ☐	Class-based behavior management program.
		☐ ☐ ☐	Fading
		☐ ☐ ☐	Biofeedback (voice-lite®)
		☐ ☐ ☐	Token Reinforcement
		☐ ☐ ☐	Other (specify)
10-3.	Did the intervention employ positive enforcement?	☐ ☐ ☐	Yes
		☐ ☐ ☐	No
		☐ ☐ ☐	Don't know
		☐ ☐ ☐	Other (specify)

NOTES:

10-4. If "yes," what was the purpose of the reinforcement procedure? [Lachenmeyer & Gibbs, 1985]

☐ ☐ ☐   To provide for incentive for the client to speak.

☐ ☐ ☐   To provide feedback to increase the clients' confidence.

☐ ☐ ☐   To provide external control of clients' behavior.

10-5. Did you play a part in the professional treatment?

☐ ☐ ☐   Yes

☐ ☐ ☐   No

10-6. If "yes," would you like to tell me about your participation?

☐ ☐ ☐

10-7. Was the professional
        treatment helpful to
        your child?

☐ ☐ ☐   Yes (explain)

☐ ☐ ☐   Somewhat (explain)

☐ ☐☐   No (explain)

NOTES:

CHAPTER 14

TREATMENT OF ELECTIVE MUTISM:
PRELIMINARY CONSIDERATIONS

JUSTIFICATION FOR TREATMENT

Sluckin (1977) comments on the importance of early treatment of elective mutism. She argues that early treatment is desirable because: (1) the educational losses will increase if electively mute children are left untreated, and (2) the children should be treated early before they learn to use silence to manipulate other people. Appelman *et al.* (1975) claimed that verbal skills are a prerequisite for much of the child's social and academic education. They also predicted developmental retardation for children lacking social skills. Lumb and Wolff (1988), however, questioned the need for intervention. They argued that:

We found it . . . very disturbing that in only one of all the reports we read [Winter cited in Lumb and Wolff, 1988] was any justification given for intervening other than that, by not speaking in certain situations, the child was deemed to have a disorder meriting intervention. Many of the interventions carried out were extremely intrusive and disruptive to the normal life of the child and family (p. 103). *Note: The study referred to is by Winter and the bibliographic details are found in Lumb and Wolff (1988).*

In their treatment guidelines, Lumb and Wolff again stressed that:

The intervention must be justified. As we noted earlier there is no general evidence that the development to adulthood of such children will be significantly impeded if no action is taken. The grounds for intervention must be clearly stated (p. 104).

They made another point which merits stating:

There should be an honest awareness that intervention will usually reflect the needs of parents and teachers rather than the needs of the child. In general children show normal academic progress and it is difficult to detect any significant enhancement of this when they begin to talk (p. 106).

Hoffman and Laub (1986) claimed that the early treatment of elective mutism increased the likelihood of the success for whatever intervention was applied to the problem. According to Furst (1989) the "education suffered" in the electively mute girl he treated. Unfortunately, his report did not elaborate on how the elective mutism negatively impacted on the child's education. Nonetheless, the successful treatment of elective mutism was correlated with above-average achievement at school.

Discussion

Referrals are often linked to the negative impacts of the mutistic response on the children's educational achievement. The published reports do not identify the area(s) of the academic or psychosocial curriculum which were impacted on negatively by the silence user role. It is, therefore, difficult to make connections between the child's beginning to speak and his or her performance in specific curriculum areas. To my knowledge, there is not a single study which systematically uses specific areas of the curriculum as dependent variable measures to assess the impact of treatment. This issue is also complicated by the fact that there is evidence for the deterioration in school performance when the child begins to talk outside the home (Weininger, 1987).

Based on a review of the work of Wilkins (1985), Bhide and Sprinath (1985) claim that there may be little justification for recognizing elective mutism as a clinical syndrome. These authors argued that shyness, anxiety and depression were features which were common among the electively mute group in the Wilkins' study. They also claimed that the Wilkins' investigation did not comment on the prevalence of transient or persistent mutism. Krolian (1988) questions whether elective mutism is a separate diagnostic entity or whether it is a symptom which cuts across a variety of diagnostic categories.

I believe that the major significance of elective mutism lies outside the elective mutism-academic performance relationship. Elective mutism can have other effects which are as important as the deterioration in academic performance. The excessive use of silence invites negative labeling and these labels may be cues for teasing or bullying. These responses in turn, could lead to the continued use of silence in order to escape or avoid these negative consequences.

RELATIONSHIP FOCUS

For electively mute individuals, establishing a therapeutic relationship rarely depends on verbal dialogue. Establishing a relationship with someone outside the family is an important component of treatment and in order for this crucial step to occur the client does not have to talk. If a therapist believes that it is necessary for the client to talk in order to establish a relationship, he or she will probably be overwhelmed by the client's silence. Furthermore, the almost exclusive focus on attempting to get a client to talk may produce a stalemate and reinforce the client's sense of power and manipulation. Kaplan and Escoll (1973) caution against waiting in silence until anxiety prompts the client to speak. These researchers advance three major arguments: (1) electively mute persons have an almost limitless capacity to tolerate silence; (2) because the client does not talk during therapy the meaning he assigns to the therapist's silence is not easily corrected or confirmed; and (3) the therapist may respond to the client with prolonged silences which serve no therapeutic function. Additional support for this position is offered by Chethik (1973); and Ruzicka and Sackin (1974) who claim that a positive treatment outcome is not necessarily equated with the child's speaking to the therapist during treatment.

Krolian (1988) identified three reasons for the positive outcome of his treatment of an electively mute adolescent: (1) an extended duration of time with the same therapist permitted the establishment of a relationship with the child; (2) the focus of therapy was on developing relationships rather than on the mutistic response; and (3) the separation from the home when the client was in the day hospital permitted him to work on the overly dependent relationship with his family. Krolian (1988) has been careful to observe and report on the context of the early speech of an electively mute child. According to the author, the child responded with single-word answers to questions while concealing himself behind a screen. The child later spoke while covering his face with a pillow. Krolian claimed that the pillow prevented the child from seeing the therapist's facial expression and this protected the child from being disappointed by any negative feedback communicated by the therapist.

My review of the literature yielded one account of a therapist who responded with silence to a three-and-a-half year old boy's silence. The therapist discontinued, however, because the child responded with immediate and prolonged screaming (Browne et al., 1963). Reed (1963) identified several strategies which are therapeutically counterproductive. Referral to a speech-language pathologist was considered counterproductive because speech and language are not ordinarily impaired in electively mute persons. Reed also cautioned against removing the patient from the family to an institutional setting. The second caution is consistent with the advantages of integrating special needs individuals into the community (Nesbit and Hadley, 1989). The only consensus about the treatment of elective mutism is that individual therapy is the least successful of interventions (Krolian, 1988). However, treating an electively mute child in a group before the child is exposed to individual therapy is a third strategy which is not recommended. But in the case of elective mutism, this may be the only option. The client may only speak in the presence of selected people and, unless they are present, may refuse to speak.

DECISION-MAKING: TOWARD LEAST RESTRICTIVE AND LEAST AVERSIVE INTERVENTIONS

Brazier and MacDonald (1981) claim that behavioral programs are sometimes designed with little consideration to positive procedures, either prior to or in combination with negative procedures (p. 11). They identified four major reasons for using positive procedures in behavior-change programs. These include:

• Positive behavior-change procedures minimize undesirable side effects such as withdrawal and aggression which are frequently associated with restrictive and aversive methods.

• Positive procedures ensure a balance between effectiveness and restrictiveness through using the least restrictive intervention in each phase of the intervention.

• Positive procedures teach the client *what to do* while restrictive and aversive methods teach the client *what not to do*. One unintended side effect of punishment is the systematic provision of a behavior control model which clients may later use in controlling the behavior of other people.

• Positive procedures involving least restrictive treatments are less likely to result in legal action and court decisions restricting the activities of behavior modifiers.

Figure 14.1 summarizes the decision-making model of Brazier and MacDonald (1981).

The interventions discussed by Brazier and MacDonald apply to behavior therapy procedures. Their model, however, is sufficiently generic to permit interventions not specified in the model to be assessed in the light of the intent of their model. Although the model was developed for institutional settings, it is also relevant for the natural environment.

There are a number of approaches which have been used alone or in combination with another therapeutic modality. Beginning at the left of Fig. 14.2, each intervention becomes progressively more intrusive. For example, play therapy and art therapy can be viewed as extending from the play of children whereas the treatments based on escape or avoidance learning are characterized by substantial therapist control.

Frequently, electively mute children are described as being "shy" and "withdrawn." The point here is to what extent does the child have the verbal and nonverbal communication skills to make talking rewarding? Directly observing the client in structured and unstructured activities and comparing the observed behavior with the verbal and nonverbal communication skills of the child's peers would answer this question.

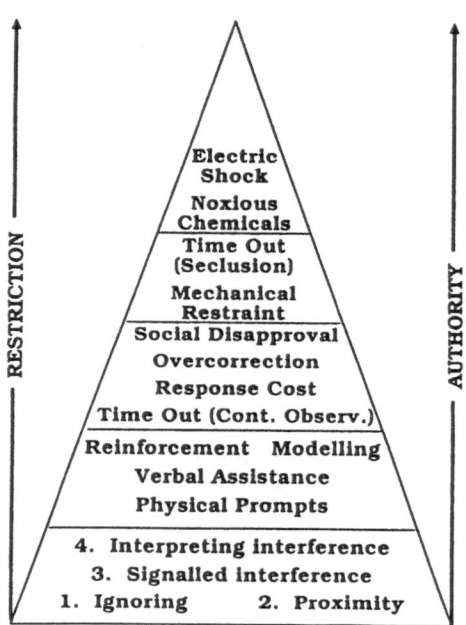

Fig. 14.1. Decision-making model based on restriction, aversion and authority.

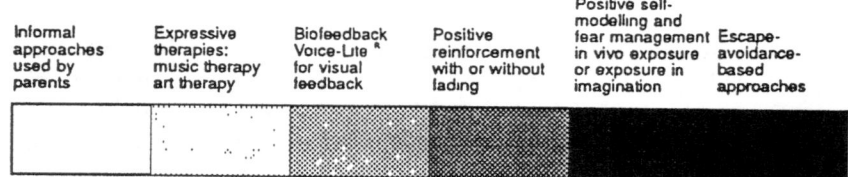

Intensity of shading represents degree of structure, intrusion and aversion

Fig. 14.2. Continuum of treatment options for elective mutism.

PROGRESSIVE MUTISM

Paniagua and Saeed (1987) added a new term, "progressive mutism," to the mental health literature. Their distinction is based on one clinical study of their own and a review of three other atypical studies of elective mutism. According to them, progressive mutism resembles elective mutism except that the children do not speak to anyone including family members. The primary characteristic of progressive mutism is that the child gradually stops talking to anyone despite the observed ability to talk and the absence of neurological and biological factors which could account for the absence of speech.

Not only have these researchers provided a useful diagnostic distinction but, in addition, they have suggested different guidelines for treating each of the two types of voluntary mutism. According to them, the focus of treatment for the electively mute child is to get him to talk to people other than close friends and family members because he already talks to these persons.

Paniagua and Saeed (1987) argued convincingly that the treatment expectations are very different for progressive mutism than for elective mutism. In the case of progressive mutism, the focus of the first phase of treatment is on getting the child to talk to family members. During this phase, there is no attempt to get the child to talk to people outside the family. The child is moved from progressive to elective mutism. Because the child now talks to family members but not to other persons, he could be described as electively rather than progressively mute. Using a single subject design, the first phase of treatment would look something like this:

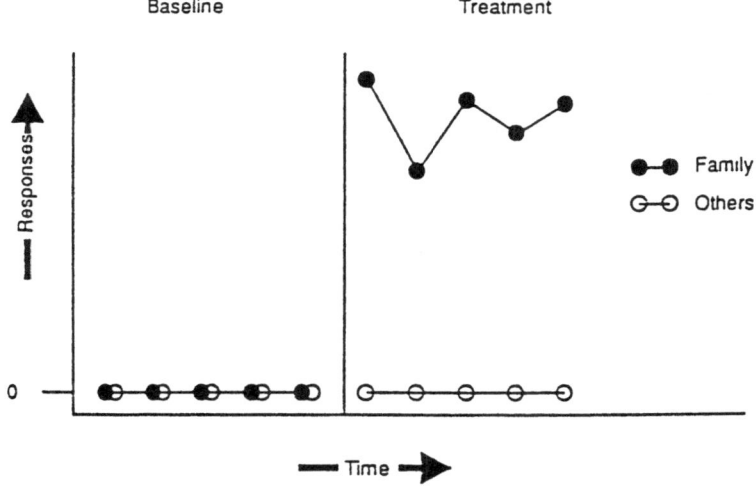

Fig. 14.3. First phase of treatment showing transition from progressive to elective mutism.

The focus of the second phase is to get the child to talk to people outside the family. Again, two baselines are collected. One baseline records the child's verbalizations within the family (●—●) and a second baseline charts the child's verbalizations with other persons (⊖—⊖). The data for phase two would look like this if the intervention was successful.

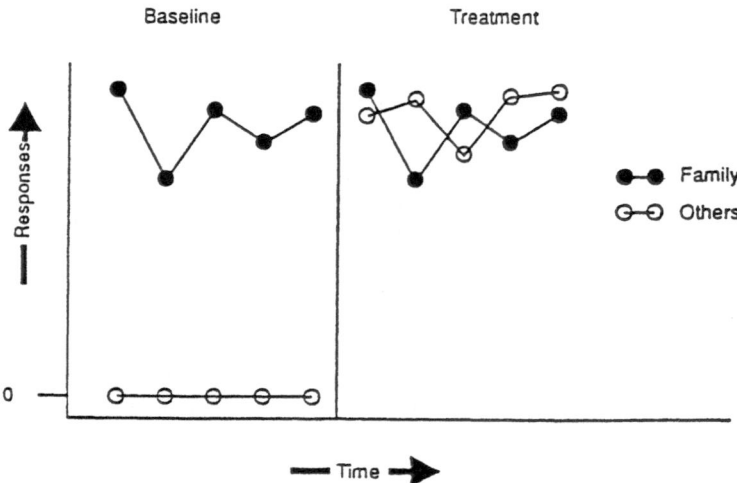

Fig. 14.4. Second phase of treatment showing transition from speech refusal to speaking to family and non-family members.

INTERVIEW STRATEGIES

Kaplan and Escoll (1973) suggest that the silent adolescent and the family be seen separately except for the diagnostic interviews early in treatment. According to them, the provocativeness of the adolescent's silence provides a ready target for scape-goating by family members. The adolescent patient and the family should be seen together when the patient and family have demonstrated readiness to relinquish the blaming communication which impedes a discussion of the family problems which may have led the client to become a silence user. Many electively mute clients begin to communicate verbally by silently mouthing words and then progress from whispering to conversational speech. The type of speech may also change from reluctant to spontaneous speech.

Table 14.1. Changes in type and volume of speech-acts.

Reluctant speech → Spontaneous speech
Silent mouthing of words → Whisper (Barely audible) → Conversational speech

The clinician should look for changes in the volume and the type of the verbal responses of the client. The previous figure outlines the sequence which is often observed during the treatment of electively mute clients.

PSYCHODYNAMIC TREATMENT

Psychodynamic treatment for elective mutism tends to last between 12–15 months and to occur in hospital/clinic settings. Treatment typically consists of play therapy with the therapist endeavoring to build up a relationship with the child. At the same time, another therapist is usually working with the parents attempting to explore and resolve family conflicts (Lumb and Wolff, 1988). Although treatment of this kind does not directly address the question of the child's silence, it nevertheless seems that the child's talking or not talking is still held to be the main indicator of success or failure in the treatment.

INSIGHT THERAPY

Insight therapy is required to deal with the attitudes, perceptions, thoughts and feelings which contributed to the individual's using silence as an expressive or coping response (Wassing, 1973). For example, if a client believed that it was necessary to be perfectly correct in everything said, the client might avoid criticism by being silent. Symptomatic treatment aimed at removing the mutistic response must precede insight therapy, however, because the client is frequently mute during the initial phases of treatment.

BEHAVIOR THERAPY

Explanations based on *learned behavior* focus more directly on teaching the child to speak in those situations where previously he or she has not done so. Indeed, interventions along behavioral lines are much more likely to be carried out in home or school with the direct involvement of parents and other children.

CRITERIA FOR RECOVERY

The therapist must determine the criteria for recovery from elective mutism. It is important to determine if an electively mute person has recovered only when he or she fails to meet DSM–III–R (or DSM–IV options) criteria. Or can less stringent criteria also constitute recovery? How long must the patient refrain from being silent in the target environment to be considered "cured?" When does a resurgence of symptoms of elective mutism indicate a relapse, as opposed to a new episode of elective mutism? By definition, recovery must delineate a stable period before a return of the symptoms could be considered a relapse. Only after that stable period of absence of speech refusal could a resurgence of symptoms be considered a recurrence. Answers to the above questions should address a number of factors. Criteria which may be helpful include: (1) the client's satisfaction with the outcome; (2) the reduction in the inconvenience to others of the client's symptom picture; (3) outcome responses as compared with baseline assessment; (4) the absence of residual symptoms; and (5) the type and magnitude of the positive impact of the behavior change on other areas of functioning of the client.

RESIDUAL SYMPTOMS

The *BASIC ID* (Lazarus, 1976) method provides a comprehensive assessment of the patient's problem because the method addresses the behavior, affect, sensations, imagery, cognitions, interpersonal relations and drugs (nutrition, sleep and health). A comprehensive assessment readily permits the identification of residual symptoms such as persistent reports of unpleasant sensations such as an upset stomach while speaking and inner statements of fear of speaking in patients who are observed to speak in settings in which they previously elected to be silent. Published reports focus on getting the client to speak in the setting in which he or she previously elected to be silent. A potential disadvantage of this approach is that the problem may have been incompletely treated for some patients. A patient can be observed to speak, yet retain the covert fear responses such as cognitions and images about speaking fears. If this occurs, the treatment has only succeeded in getting the child to exhibit courage. Effective treatment necessitates monitoring dependent variable measures based on the BASIC ID (Lazarus, 1976) during baseline, treatment and follow-up.

CHAPTER 15

EARLIEST COMMUNICATION DURING TREATMENT
OF ELECTIVELY MUTE PERSONS

EARLIEST COMMUNICATION

I have carefully reviewed a number of research studies to determine the earliest communication of electively mute individuals during treatment. There were, however, a few studies in which the first communication was either not reported or was reported in such a way that it was difficult to determine when it occurred during therapy (e.g., "after Phase 1" or during the "later stages of treatment"). In the absence of more precise information, this data was included because it indicated if the first communication occurred in the beginning, middle or in the final phase of treatment. In several of the studies, it was difficult to identify the treatment modality and it was therefore necessary to decide on a description which closely approximated the researcher's intervention (e.g., "play therapy" for finger painting and doll play).

Table 15.1. Earliest communication of electively mute individuals during treatment.

Research study	Method of treatment	Description of earliest communication(s)	Onset of earliest communication(s)
Salfield (1950)	Play Therapy	Answered questions in mono-syllables when coaxed	6th month
Morris (1953)	Play Therapy	Case 1: Yes/no responses to questions	Not reported
	Play Therapy	Case 2: Spoke in whispers, but no reaction to noise or music	6th month
	Play Therapy	Case 3: Spoke a few words in a whisper	Not reported
Parker, Olsen, & Throckmorton (1960)	Use of orifices and clay, mouthing of sounds and words	Case 1: Spoke while facing clinician's back	2nd session
Mora, DeVault, & Schopler (1962)	Art and Play Therapy	*Twins:* Written communication	After Phase 1

149

Table 15.1. (Continued).

Research study	Method of treatment	Description of earliest communication(s)	Onset of earliest communication(s)
Reed (1963)	Re-learning for all 4 cases	Case 1: Monosyllabic responses	After a few sessions
		Case 3: Monosyllabic responses to direct questions	Not reported
		Case 4: Monosyllabic responses	Not reported
Browne, Wilson, & Laybourne (1963)	Play Therapy	Animal sounds and yes/no responses during client's self occlusion of vision (head in wastebasket)	Not reported
Elson, Pearson, Jones, & Schumacher (1965)	Psychotherapy and art therapy	Spoke freely to all children even in presence of hospital staff	7th month
Nolan & Pence (1970)	Positive reinforcement contingency	Whispering elicited by prompts	4th day
Norman & Broman (1970)	Positive reinforcement (visual feedback from the volume-level meter of a tape recorder)	Smiled and made a low sound	1st session
Wassing (1970)	Positively reinforced successive approximations	Whispered softly into a tape recorder	End of 2nd session
Halpern, Hammond, & Cohen (1971)	Behavior modification using graded approach	Whispered the word "go"	Not reported
Chethik (1973)	Art Therapy (working with clay, "scissors work and drawing"), play therapy, story-telling,"talking folder" in anticipation of child's talking	Took therapist's hand while walking to therapy setting	1st session
Dmitriev & Hawkins (1973)	Positive reinforcement contingency	One word responses	5th day of treatment
Marcus, Holt, & Nagurney (1973)	Positive reinforcement for carrying out errands	Case 1: Spoke at the school office while on an errand	Not reported
	Audio-taping personal interests and hobbies of all students	Case 2: Verbal statements on a tape recorder	Not reported

Table 15.1. (Continued).

Research study	Method of treatment	Description of earliest communication(s)	Onset of earliest communication(s)
Pustrom & Speers (1964)	Art Therapy (finger-painting)	Case 1: Spoke in the waiting room but not to therapist during treatment	Later stages of treatment
	Finger-painting and doll play	Case 3: Did not speak to therapist during treatment, but spoke to her teacher and other female adults	Later stages of treatment
Rosenbaum & Kellman (1973)	Shaping	Spoke when prompted	Phase 1
Reid, Hawkins, Keutzer, McNeal, Phelps, Reid, & Mees (1973)	Reinforcement and stimulus fading	Spoke to a stranger without looking at him	Stage 3
Ayllon & Kelly (1974)	Operant conditioning	Verbal responses, when shaped outside the classroom	Session 8
Bednar (1974)	Operant conditioning using immediate positive reinforcement	"Clicking sound" prompted by offer of a penny	Beginning of 6th session
Conrad, Delk, & Williams (1974)	Stimulus fading	Verbally responded to flashcards	1st treatment at home
Rasbury (1974)	In vivo desensitization with positive reinforcement in the client's natural environment	Spontaneous speech to non-family members	Final phase
Ruzicka & Sackin (1974)	Game play	Participation in a game of Chutes 'n' Ladders	Late stages of treatment
Wulbert, Nyman, Snow, & Owen (1973)	Stimulus fading and contingency management	Responded verbally	Day 7
Bauermeister & Jemail (1975)	Operant conditioning	Answered questions and read aloud to therapist	Phase 3
Landgarten (1975)	Art Therapy	Occasionally said a few words, (e.g., titles for paint dabs and ambiguous collages)	1st month
Van der Kooy & Webster (1975)	Avoidance conditioning under water	Said "no" to avoid aversive stimulus of being dunked	4th week
Colligan, Colligan, & Dilliard (1977)	Operant reinforcement and contingency management techniques	Nonverbal communication (unspecified) with teacher	1st three weeks

Table 15.1. (Continued).

Research study	Method of treatment	Description of earliest communication(s)	Onset of earliest communication(s)
Radford (1977)	Psychotherapy – Play and Art	Spoke to therapist	Later sessions
Sluckin (1977)	Shaping of speaking into a tape recorder	Case 1: Verbally told clinician how to locate his home	Beginning of treatment
		Case 2: Spoke to other children	
Williamson, Sanders, Sewell, Haney & White (1977)	Shaping with modeling	Case 1 & 2: Imitation of blowing	2nd session
Crema & Kerr (1978)	Empathetic approach and stimulus fading	Spoke to therapist	During 1st month
Richards & Hansen (1978)	Stimulus fading beginning in the environment where the client spoke and through approximations to where the client did not talk	Spoke in whispers, one word responses and occasionally short answers	1st 5 sessions
Rosenberg & Lindblad (1978)	Reinforcement with telephone used as a medium	Spoke in single words	Phase 1
Ambrosino & Alessi (1979)	Triadic setting – male psychiatrist, female psychologist and child. Token reinforcement	Gestures, nodding head, and a guttural/snorting sound, spoke into a tape recorder when alone	Beginning of therapy
Nash, Thorpe, Andrews, & Davis (1979)	Operant shaping	Case 1: Made the "h" sound	3rd day: 195th command
	Operant shaping	Case 2: Made the "h" sound	
	Negative reinforcement	Case 3: Spoke the word "yes"	
Youngerman (1979)	Operant conditioning	Case 1: Spoke to psychologist	Unknown
		Case 2: A "frighteningly demonic grin"	After several weeks
Blotcky & Looney (1980)	Behavioral play therapy	Spoke freely	6th month

Table 15.1. (Continued).

Research study	Method of treatment	Description of earliest communication(s)	Onset of earliest communication(s)
Lipton (1980)	Biofeedback progressively louder volume required to move string	Child whispered more than three words in response to questions	5th session
Clayton (1981)	Stimulus fading and positive reinforcement	Silently mouthed words	1st session
Heimlich (1981)	Peer counselling	Spoke phrase to peer counsellor	1st session
Kupietz & Schwartz (1982)	Stimulus fading	Case 1: Speaking in mother's presence while at school	2nd month of treatment
	Stimulus fading	Case 2: Spoke with his father in normal conversational voice during learning activities at school	After eight sessions
	Stimulus fading	Case 3: Whispered to his mother in teacher's presence	14th session
Morin, Ladouceur, & Cloutier (1982)	Reinforcement contingency procedure	Verbally responded to questions. Initially treatment conducted outside the classroom (teacher + 2 children) led client to talk	5th session, Phase B
Subak, West, & Carlin (1982)	Informal – walking, game words playing, (penny arcade downtown)	Laughing, speaking one or two words	Not reported
Cunningham, Cataldo, Mallion, & Keyes (1983)	Play Therapy	Case 1: Spoke to teacher during individual play therapy	Early in treatment
	Positively reinforced for imitating responses	Case 2: Imitation of nonverbal responses	Sessions 1–3
Sluzki (1983)	Family Therapy	Case 1: Nodding to the therapist's request to teach English to her "father." At the close of the session "the daughter broke her silence and uttered with animation to the therapist, 'Do you like my new overcoat? I got it for my birthday a week ago.'"	1st session
		Case 2: Speaking associated with transfer to new school	3 months

Table 15.1. (Continued).

Research study	Method of treatment	Description of earliest communication(s)	Onset of earliest communication(s)
Zondlo & Scanlan (1983)	26-day hospitalization. [This client was profoundly deaf.]	Spoke in response to the staff's attempts at conversation. Speech was unintelligible except for the word "no."	Not reported
Bozigar & Hansen (1984)	Group Play Therapy [toy animals, storytelling, and tape recorders]	Hello and good-bye by touching, shaking hands, or waving	Early stages
Ciottone & Madonna (1984)	Combination of group play therapy and videotaped playback	Written work on a board (doing and correcting mathematics problems)	Not reported
Roberts (1984)	Family Therapy: Haley Strategic Model and Milan Model	Writing with correct grammar and spelling	Not reported
Coutts (1985)	Desensitization program	Monosyllabic answers in a husky voice	Not reported
Harvey, Green, & Newton (1985)	Token reinforcement	Spoke a few spontaneous words to a nurse	Shortly after 10 weeks
Hill & Scull (1985)	Positive reinforcement	Silently mouthed words during reading	Approximately 2 months
Lachenmeyer & Gibbs (1985)	Reinforcement contingency procedure	Reinforcement contingent on brief verbal response to questions. Client immediately responded verbally.	1st session with teacher as therapist
Southworth (1985)	Tape recording the client's reading	Whispered in teacher's ear	3rd month
Winter (1985)	Contingent reinforcement	Two utterances per day in school	1st week
Winter (1985)	Contingency reinforcement	Spoke spontaneously in words, phrases and sentences	4th week
Wright, Miller, Cook, & Littmann (1985)	Play at a nursery program	Case 1: Spoke spontaneously while playing outside	3rd week
		Case 2: One or two word labelling	2nd week
		Case 3: One or two words to peers	1st day

Table 15.1. (Continued).

Research study	Method of treatment	Description of earliest communication(s)	Onset of earliest communication(s)
Albert-Stewart (1986)	Shaping of voice volume and speech intelligibility	Short sentences, monotone, voice so low, difficult to hear	First individual therapy session
Barlow, Strother, & Landreth (1986)	Play Therapy	Gestured in 1st session, spoke with friend during 2nd session	1st & 2nd session
Hoffman & Laub (1986)	Paradoxical therapy in the context of a polarization model of co-therapy with behavioral techniques in a family therapy framework	Indirect verbal communication with therapists through the client's brother – "The psychologist is an idiot."	Not reported
Beck & Hubbard (1987)	Expressive Therapy	A hug during a client-initiated game of hide and seek	Early stages of therapy
Paniagua & Saeed (1987)	Response-cost and correct imitations were followed by praise	Named three picture cards (cat, car, telephone)	4th session
Pigott & Gonzales (1987)	Playroom observation	Curled up in fetal position in response to therapist questions – answered questions by writing	Assessment phase
Weininger (1987)	Play Therapy	Case 1: After 4 weeks of twice a week sessions, spoke – "The poo stays in the toilet." Case 2: Non-verbal communication nodded "yes" and did three drawings	4 weeks
Krolian (1988)	Individual, Group and Art Therapy	Case 1: Used sign language to communicate with classmates and teacher	1 year
	Milieu therapy at day hospital	Case 2: Whispering to 12-year-old patient. Escaped from tickling or pinching by speaking	1st week after admission
Brown & Doll (1988)	Play Therapy: Classroom based behavior management program	Spoke to classmates when prompted	1st day of treatment
Lesser-Katz (1988)	Play Therapy	Nodded in answer to a question	3rd session

Table 15.1. (Continued).

Research study	Method of treatment	Description of earliest communication(s)	Onset of earliest communication(s)
Carr & Afnan (1989)	Concurrent individual play therapy and family therapy	Whispered to her mother in school	After 3rd family therapy session and 5th play therapy session
Furst (1989)	Contingent reinforce-ment during game play	Client replied, "You have to pick up three cards from the card bank," in response to physician's statement that he did not know the rules of the game.	First occasion of game play following one home consultation and four one-half hour weekly clinic meetings
Kehle, Owen, & Cressey (1990)	Self-modeling answering teacher's questions	Spontaneously spoke to therapists	2nd day of intervention while observing inter-vention videotape

Table 15.1 indicates that behavior therapy was the treatment of choice in the majority of the studies. Defined contingencies with positive reinforcing consequences were the typical behavior therapy employed in treating elective mutism. In a number of studies elective mutism seems to have been equated with speech phobia. Various types of gestures are reported as being the first observable communication of the client during therapy. Prosocial gestures which marked the first communication to occur during therapy included smiling (Norman and Broman, 1970), participation in a board game (Ruzicka and Sackin, 1974), unspecified nonverbal communication with a teacher (Colligan *et al.*, 1977), nodding head in response to questions (Ambrosino and Alessi, 1979; Lesser-Katz, 1988), unspecified gestures (Barlow *et al.*, 1986), and communicating "hello" and "goodbye" by shaking hands, touching, or waving (Bozigar and Hansen, 1984).

Of the forms of communication to occur first, whispering was the second most frequent. Whispering as a first observable communication was reported by Morris (1953), Nolan and Pence (1970), Wassing (1970), Halpern *et al.* (1971), Richards and Hansen (1978), Kupietz and Schwartz (1982), Southworth (1985), Barrett and Krolian (1988), and Carr and Afnan (1989).

Spontaneous vocalization of specific sounds or imitation of specific sounds ranked third. Bednar (1974) reported the occurrence of a "clicking sound;" Williamson *et al.* (1977) observed the imitation of a blowing sound; Ambrosino and Alessi (1979) reported a guttural-snorting sound; Nash *et al.* (1979) indicated that they succeeded in getting their client to imitate the "h" sound. Browne *et al.* (1963) observed that their client made animal sounds while putting his head in a waste basket in order to occlude his vision and avoid eye contact with the therapist.

The fourth most frequent form of first communication was spontaneous speech. Unfortunately, the researchers do not define spontaneous speech but presumably it includes the verbal communication which occurs independent of therapists' questions or prompting. Rasbury (1974) reported spontaneous speech to non-family members; Blotcky and Looney (1980) claimed that their client spoke freely during play therapy while Harvey *et al.* (1985) asserted that their client voluntarily said a few words to a nurse. Winter (1985) indicated that his client spoke spontaneously in words, phrases and sentences, and Wright *et al.* (1985) said that one of their clients spontaneously spoke while playing outside.

Other low frequency first communication responses to occur were also identified. Silent mouthing of words was reported by Hill and Scull (1985) and Clayton (1981). Verbal responses which were infrequently reported in the literature were "yes" or "no" (Brown *et al.*, 1963; Nash *et al.*, 1979; Zondlo and Scanlan, 1983). Monosyllabic and one-word responses were mentioned by Coutts (1985); Reed, (1963); Halpern *et al.* (1971); Van der Kooy and Webster (1975); Rosenberg and Lindblad (1978); Salfield, (1950); and Wright *et al.* (1985). Only the research of Mora *et al.* (1962) and Roberts (1984) identified written communication as the first step toward verbal communication.

Discussion

It must be recognized that the topography of the responses which occur early in treatment depend not only on the motivations and preferences of the silence users but also on the instructions of the therapist. For example, if a therapist instructed the client to respond by nodding his head for "Yes" or moving his head from side-to-side for "No," the client would probably be more inclined to communicate nonverbally, rather than to use other communication responses.

Rarely do descriptions of the pretreatment status or progress reports during treatment include data on the client's use of nonverbal behavior. In fact, there are no studies that I am aware of which deal with the nonverbal communication of electively mute persons. This would make a fascinating topic for an enterprising postgraduate student. Nonetheless, several studies (Colligan *et al.*, 1977; Ambrosino and Alessi, 1979; Clayton, 1981; Hill and Skull, 1985; Barlow *et al.*, 1986; Beck and Hubbard, 1987; Pigott and Gonzales, 1987; Weininger, 1987; Barrett and Krolian, 1988) reported that a nonverbal response was the client's first observed communication. Nonverbal communication seemed to have been considered of minimal importance because the target of the treatment was verbal behavior. Questions left unanswered include the following: Did the gestures which were observed before treatment differ from those which were observed during treatment? and, if so, how were they modified or amplified? When spontaneous speech is reported, it involves highly structured situations, such as "Tell me a story about what is happening in the picture," rather than of spontaneous speech involving the initiation of dialogue.

Table 15.1 reveals that typically early communication responses were whispering, nonverbal responses such as nodding "Yes," or one or two word responses. The majority of these responses, however, occurred after being prompted by a therapist or mediator. Rarely did electively mute children not begin to talk in the target setting after being in treatment for six months. Studies employing expressive therapy approaches either alone or in combination with behavior therapy procedures addressed the relationship aspect of communication in addition to eliciting speech from electively mute persons.

CHAPTER 16

FOLLOW-UP OF ELECTIVELY MUTE PERSONS

FOLLOW-UP REPORTS

The follow-up reports of individuals treated for elective mutism are presented in Table 16.1. The practical constraints on clinical work do not make it easy to include a formal follow-up evaluation. The preparation of the table was complicated because a number of studies did not indicate the method of assessing the status of the client. Reports of the follow-up phases frequently amount to anecdotal reports rather than clearly defined dependent variable measures such as the duration of speaking, and the number or frequency of words spoken. Unfortunately, the majority of the anecdotal reports do not clearly indicate if the client spoke only when asked a question (reluctant speech) or if the person voluntarily contributed to conversations (spontaneous speech). Evidence of advance planning for a systematic follow-up is absent in the majority of the studies. A systematic follow-up should specify the method of obtaining information (telephone or face-to-face interview, questionnaire or direct observation by the investigator) as well as the questions which were employed. It is also advisable to include the same dependent variables in the follow-up assessment that were employed in assessing the internal validity of the intervention. Client satisfaction with treatment is one additional measure of treatment effectiveness but studies rarely address this issue either at the conclusion of treatment or at follow-up.

Table 16.1. Studies reporting follow-up of electively mute persons.

Research study	Method	Time between treatment and follow-up	Comments
Morris (1953) N = 6	Informal monitoring	Not stated	One case – unimproved; 4 out of 6 showed satisfactory improvement; one case – no information
Parker, Olsen, & Throckmorton (1960)	Report by mother	Not stated	Client spoke freely with no evidence of any prior difficulty in communicating

Table 16.1. (Continued).

Research study	Method	Time between treatment and follow-up	Comments
Reed (1963) N = 4	Unspecified	Approximately 3–5 years	3 of 4 cases showed speech maintenance, while one case remained silent but better adapted to community living
Browne, Wilson, & Laybourne (1963)	Report by teacher	Not stated	Client was talking in corridors and in line where speech was forbidden
Elson, Pearson, Jones & Schumacher (1965) N = 4	One interview for each of 4 girls and their mothers, using a revised form of a Follow-up Coding Manual devised by Dr. Peter Beckett of the Lafayette Clinic.	5 years (duration of 6 months)	Significant improvement in talking to friends and strangers
Nolan & Pence (1970)	Evaluation by senior author with the family in their home	1 year	Speech was indistinguishable from classmates
Norman & Broman (1970)	Report by peers, & PTA member	18 months	Speaking outside the home. Routinely answers telephone at home and progressed from simple "yes–no" statements to complete sentences.
Wassing (1970)	Report by client	Over a year	Speaking in school and elsewhere
Halpern, Hammond, & Cohen (1971)	Report by teacher	Immediately after	Twins asked questions, talked to teachers and occasionally in class
Dmitriev & Hawkins (1973)	Report by teacher	Unspecified	Doing well academically and actively involved in Girl Scouts
Marcus, Holt, & Nagurney (1973) N = 2	Observation by teacher	Not specified, but appears to be directly after treatment	Both cases improved academically and socially
Pustrom & Spears (1964) N=4	1 of the 4 cases: Report by mother via letter	Unspecified	General improvement in all 4 cases, although none talked to the therapist
Rosenbaum & Kellman (1973)	Report by teacher	2–1/2 months	Participating fully in all class activities

Table 16.1. (Continued).

Research study	Method	Time between treatment and follow-up	Comments
Reid, Hawkins, Keitzer, McNeal, Phelps, Reid, & Mees (1973)	3 meetings at the clinic, and report by mother	2 weeks	Client was verbalizing freely outside the clinic
Ayllon & Kelly (1974)	Observation sessions, 15 minutes in length, by an assistant unknown to client. Responses were recorded verbatim, in 3 different sessions with 3 different teachers.	1 year	Evidence of spontaneous speech; two new teachers were surprised to hear that the child had been electively mute.
Bednar (1974)	Report by school counselor and one interview (identity of interviewer not specified)	2 years	Spontaneous speech with teachers and pupils
Conrad, Delk, & Williams (1974)	Parental interview by a female paraprofessional in client's home	1 year	Routinely talks in classroom
Bauermeister & Jemail (1975)	Unspecified	1 year	Child still talking in classroom
Landgarten (1975) N = 2	Case 1: Informal report by teacher	2 months after mother prematurely terminated treatment	Child continued to express herself through drawings and collages but did not speak at the conclusion of therapy or at follow-up.
	Case 2: Informal report initiated by father	Report at 6 months	Indications of rapid regression, possibly due to abandonment of family by mother
Van der Kooy, & Webster (1975)	Informal report by teacher	6 months, at end of summer vacation	Speaking appropriately in social situations and at school
Colligan, Colligan, & Dilliard (1977)	Teacher report based on two home visits	1 year	Quality and frequency of speech maintained
Sluckin (1977) N = 2	Case 1: Report by headmistress, class teacher, and mother	6 months	Progress both academically and socially. Boisterous and eager to learn; talked to all visitors in the home
	Case 2: Report by social worker	2 months	Communicating normally both in the playground and classroom

Table 16.1. (Continued).

Research study	Method	Time between treatment and follow-up	Comments
Williamson, Sanders, Sewell, Haney & White (1977) N = 2	Case 1: Teacher interview	2 weeks	Speaking normally in class including one recitation to class
	Case 1: Teacher interview	1 year	Responded to all questions from teacher and peers, and occasionally spoke spontaneously in class
	Case 2: Teacher interview, prompts to read were reintroduced for 3 sessions	1 month	Responded verbally without reinforcement to all requests in all classes
Crema & Kerr (1978)	Follow-up of verbal performance continued for 4 weeks. Assessments included mother and school personnel.	Immediately after treatment	Absence of verbal difficulties
Richards & Hansen (1978)	Unspecified	15 months and at 5 years	Continued to speak in school and progressed normally in academic work
Rosenberg & Lindblad (1978)	Report by school counselor	1–1/2 years	Excellent progress in regular classroom
		6 years (Same client)	Satisfactory adjustment to junior high
Ambrosino & Alessi (1979)	Report by client's 2 therapists	1 year	Spoke spontaneously to both therapists
Nash, Thorpe, Andrews, & Davis (1979) N = 3	Case 1: Observation by two raters, simultaneously and independently, preceded by one hour of training in making ratings based on observations	2 years	Verbal compliance and self-initiated comments
	Case 2: Same as #1	2 years	Verbally non-compliant
	Case 3: Same as #1	1 year	During 30-minute time frame, there were 17 instances of verbal compliance, plus two self-initiated comments.
Sanok & Ascoine (1979)	Discussion with teachers supported parental report	10 months	Verbal in all classes, but no increase in spontaneous speech

Table 16.1. (Continued).

Research study	Method	Time between treatment and follow-up	Comments
Lipton (1980)	Reports from teachers and parents	6 months	Spoke freely with no recurrence of mutism
Clayton (1981)	Independent reports from peers, and playground observation by the psychologist	9 months	Spoke spontaneously with pupils and staff
Heimlich (1981)	Report by mother and teachers	Not specified	Spoke to peers and adults
Morin, Ladouceur, & Cloutier (1982)	Direct observation by teacher and another observer	1 year	Therapeutic benefits maintained at optimal level. Child spontaneously spoke and answered questions.
Kupietz & Schwartz (1982) N = 3	No follow-up reported for Cases 1 and 2, direct observation for Case 3 (nine-year-old male)	Unclear	Case 3: Talked to examiner in a quiet subdued voice and wrote his name on request
Sluzki (1983) N = 2	Family A: First follow-up unspecified	3 months	Initially too talkative and violent with other children but that also subsided
	Family A: Second follow-up; method unspecified	6 months	No new problems in any family member
	Family B: First follow-up telephone interview	3 months	Doing fine and quite talkative
	Family B: Second follow-up unspecified	6 months	As above for 3 month follow-up
Zondlo & Scanlan (1983) N = 2	Case 1: Personnel from residential life-skills facility for deaf adults	Immediately following hospitalization	Hospitalized for aggressive behaviors
	Case 2: Personnel from residential facility for deaf adults	8 months	Communication is improved. No episodes of aggressive or psychotic behavior
Cunningham, Cataldo, Mallion, & Keyes (1983) N = 2	Case 1: Parents and teacher independently reported progress	6 months	Speaking with peers and adults at home and school
	Case 2: Telephone interview with client and family	1 and 2 months	Parents noted that he spoke consistently at school and to other children
Bozigar & Hansen (1984) N = 4	Report by teachers	3 months, 6 months, and one year	All four children were symptom free

Table 16.1. (Continued).

Research study	Method	Time between treatment and follow-up	Comments
Ciottone & Madonna (1984)	Direct observation of child on the playground	Beginning of the following school year – preceded by 20 treatment sessions	Observed talking and initiating play with other children
Roberts (1984)	Informal	Not stated	Improvement in integration with society (good grades, making new friends and joining the choir)
Harvey, Green, & Newton (1985)	Unspecified	Seven months	Quality of verbal and nonverbal communication improved
Lachenmeyer & Gibbs (1985)	Reports from parents and teachers	1 year	No special problems that would single the client out in class. Initiated conversations with adults to whom he had previously not spoken.
Winter (1985)	Reynell Scale, and behavioral observation	2 months and 1 year	Expressive language age had improved by the 6th month of therapy. General improvement in social skills
Albert-Stewart (1986)	Report by teacher	Not stated	Infrequent, mild remissions were followed by prompt resumption of therapeutic gains on the same or following day
Atoynatan (1986)	Case 1: Unspecified	Not stated	'No recurrence of the mutism'
	Case 2: Unspecified	2 years	Relinquished her mutism and no problem in speaking with men
Hoffman & Laub (1986)	Parental report	2 months	Spoke to an increasing number of people; expanded her circle of friends in kindergarten. Age appropriate behavior.
Beck & Hubbard (1987)	Client-initiated correspondence to therapist	Shortly after treatment, and again at 24 months	Client had moved to Africa and had made new friends. Progressing well academically and was relating well to adults and children

Table 16.1. (Continued).

Research study	Method	Time between treatment and follow-up	Comments
Pigott & Gonzales (1987)	Telephone follow-up report by mother	6 months	Improvement – "straight A's in school" – talked in class and with classmates over the telephone
Weininger (1987) N = 2	Case 1: Unspecified	4 months	Subject continued talking; no further problems.
	Case 2: Follow-up not available		Children developed other problems; reading difficulties, somatic complaints, depression.
Lesser-Katz (1988) N = 15	Unspecified	Several assessments over a three-year period	Each of 15 clients continued to speak and were doing well academically.
Furst (1989)	Unspecified	2 years following treatment	Client conversed with everyone and was above average achiever.
Crumley (1990)	Contacted periodically by telephone and interviewed with parents at age 29	20 years	Currently avoids crowds and talking to people in small spaces
Kehle, Owen & Cressey (1990)	Direct observation and reports from peers and school personnel	7 months	Communicated freely with peers and faculty. Volunteered to assist authors with other mute children

Table 16.1 indicates that parents were typically the informants for the follow-up evaluations. The rationale for using parents is not clear because ordinarily the home is one setting in which the client elects to talk and one would not expect to see substantial changes in the verbal behavior of the client in this setting either at the conclusion of treatment or at follow-up. In fact, parents are often surprised to learn, at the time of referral, that their son or daughter does not talk in the target setting.

In two studies (Norman and Broman, 1970; Kehle *et al.*, 1990), the researchers indicated that peers served as informants in the follow-up assessment of the previously electively mute person. In Crumley's (1990) 20-year follow-up investigation and in two other studies (Elson *et al.*, 1965; Wassing, 1970), the clients were interviewed about the status of their verbal behavior. Beck and Hubbard (1987) obtained follow-up information from client-initiated correspondence with the therapist. In several other studies

(Marcus *et al.*, 1973; Ayllon and Kelly, 1974; Nash *et al.*, 1979; Clayton, 1981; Kupietz and Schwartz, 1982; Kehle *et al.*, 1990), however, direct observation was the primary source of the follow-up data.

Of the studies reviewed, only two clients were described as unimproved at follow-up. Only one patient (Weininger, 1987) developed other learning and behavior problems (reading difficulties, somatic complaints and depression) which coincided with the onset of the client's speaking in the target setting. Table 16.1, therefore, suggests that (1) a wide variety of treatments are successful in treating the target behavior problem of speech refusal and (2) clinicians have reason to be optimistic about the prognosis for elective mutism.

EXPLANATIONS FOR BECOMING A SILENCE USER

The report by Colligan *et al.* (1977) is one of the few studies which discusses the client's explanation for electing to become a silence user. These researchers asked their client at the conclusion of treatment why he elected to become a silence user. The client's statement, "I can't understand why I didn't talk before," suggests that the client was either unwilling or unable to discuss the attitudes and perceptions which may have influenced him to become a silence user. Insight therapy, however, did not follow symptomatic treatment and hence additional information is unavailable. Hoffman and Laub (1986) also addressed this question. They asserted that the four-and-a-half-year old kindergarten girl claimed that "the reason that she did not speak to adults in the past was that she had a sore throat and last week it stopped hurting" (p. 141).

The six-year-old female client of Carr and Afnan (1989) presented a detailed retrospective account of her speech refusal. The female client believed that her mother wanted her to remain mute so that she could come to school and speak for her. The young client saw herself as inadequate and incompetent. The authors claimed that it was these beliefs that prevented her from speaking in challenging and unfamiliar activities. The client was unable to differentiate between feelings of sadness and anger in herself and others, although she could identify happiness and fear.

At the conclusion of treatment a six-year-old boy in the Kehle *et al.* (1990) research answered questions about himself but his response to the question, "Why did you not talk?" was "I don't remember not talking." Although symptomatic treatment was successful, it seems that the child was unable or unwilling to verbalize his reasons for electing to be silent. The self-modeling intervention used by Kehle *et al.* (1990) succeeded in getting the child to talk. The change in behavior was clearly demonstrated in a number of ways including the child's answering questions about himself. The treatment objectives, however, did not include obtaining detailed retrospective accounts of the reasons for the child's electing to be silent. Furthermore, identifying and correcting self-defeating philosophies about speaking in public were not a focus of the intervention. Therefore, it is not surprising that the child responded the way he did to the question. Identifying and correcting self-defeating cognitions and dysfunctional family rules depends on dialogue and the patient's emitting verbal behavior precedes examining and modifying dysfunctional cognitions and communication stances.

An equally important question is, "Why did the client commence talking?" This question has been indirectly addressed in studies which provided evidence for the internal validity of their investigations. The question "Is the intervention responsible for getting the child to talk?" does not address the lived experience of the patient. It is not the same as asking, "Why did you commence talking?" Except for the Krolian (1988) report, I do not know of a single investigation in which the patient was asked why he or she began to talk to the therapist and to others outside the context of therapy. The study reported asking the client why *she started to talk* to the therapist. Krolian's young client replied that "We'll talk about that in two weeks." Unfortunately, the author did not report the client's delayed response to his query.

Discussion

The majority of studies do not ask the client (or an informant) before, during, or after treatment why she or he elected to be silent in the target setting. It is appreciated that this question is subject to retrospective recall. I am referring to the tendency of clients to modify their account of the acquisition of their problem to coincide with the treatment outcome (Robins, 1966). A BASIC ID behavioral analysis (Lazarus, 1976) is recommended because it permits a comprehensive retrospective account to be obtained on this important issue. I predict that if the assessment and treatment addressed behavior, affect, sensation, imagery, cognition, interpersonal relations, and drugs (nutrition, sleep and health), it is likely that the retrospective account would be more comprehensive and accurate than requests for information which focus on the speech-act. There is, however, another class of equally important questions which have been addressed in only one study (Krolian, 1988). This class of questions relate to why the client spoke to the therapist and to others in the setting which was previously associated with speech-refusal. Answers to this class of questions are important because they not only improve our understanding of elective mutism but, in addition, they may illuminate important therapeutic factors.

REACTIONS TO IMPROVEMENT

When the parents of an eight-year boy discovered that he was talking freely at the day hospital, they refused to keep a single appointment. Krolian (1988) reasoned that the family felt that their son was doing so well that he did not require further treatment. Krolian also claimed that the family experienced their son's verbal talkativeness as an abandonment and rejection of their closed family system.

CHAPTER 17

UNSYSTEMATIC INFORMAL TREATMENTS

METHODS USED BY PARENTS

Parents may show little motivation to get their child to talk in settings outside the home because the child does talk to family members. Because the child does talk at home and, perhaps, even outside the home in the presence of the parents, they may find it hard to believe that their child is a silence user. Parents who are inclined to believe that their child is electively mute frequently attempt to elicit speech by using both positive and negative strategies. A commonly used positive method involves offering a variety of gifts, but negative methods are also frequently employed and include:
- badgering the child,
- embarrassing the child for not talking in the presence of strangers,
- removing privileges and administering punishment such as withdrawing meals,
- ignoring the child by withdrawing verbal communication, and
- accompanying the child to the classroom but leaving when the child's back is turned (Pustrom and Speers, 1964).

Generally, parental attempts at treatment are unsuccessful. Negative methods may even inadvertently reinforce the mutism because of the increased attention which the child receives when these tactics are applied. Nonetheless, the escape training used by the twelve year old peer (tickling until the electively mute female said "I love you") succeeded in getting the electively mute child to emit a three word prosocial response (Krolian, 1988).

Freidman and Karagan (1973) identified three potentially helpful interventions that parents can use with an electively mute child. These include: (1) involving the child in story-telling and other verbal activities, (2) including the child in a variety of peer activities in a number of different settings, and (3) encouraging the child's relatives and peers to visit the home so that the electively mute child will have an opportunity to speak in their presence.

SPEECH SETTING OF THE SILENCE USER

I prefer a booth in a restaurant because it provides a more intimate atmosphere than other seating arrangements. Another reason, is that it is more comfortable and this in turn might contribute to relaxed communication. Setting preferences, however, are rarely included in an assessment of speech refusal, yet this information would be useful in planning least restrictive treatments.

Little is known about how electively mute individuals perceive the physical setting and people to whom they elect not to talk. Furthermore, the impact of their perceptions on the target problem has not been the subject of a psychological study. This is not surprising, however, because electively mute clients frequently do not speak during treatment although preliminary information about the impact of the physical environment could be readily obtained from family members with whom the individual speaks. The question about how the setting has changed or is perceived to have changed during or after treatment is also left unanswered. Environmental psychology demonstrates that the physical setting influences communication (Bell *et al.*, 1990). An important feature of elective mutism is that the person talks in one setting but not in another. In spite of this well accepted characteristic, a description of the setting or the potential impact of the physical setting on verbal communication is rarely included in the assessment of electively mute behavior. Another equally important issue is that we do not know about the physical characteristics of the setting which may contribute to the ease of communication for speech refusal.

Treatments of elective mutism almost exclusively focus on symptomatic treatment. Very little information is provided about the physical characteristics of a setting which is associated with the problem of speech refusal. Elaborate descriptions are provided, however, of the characteristics of the electively mute person including the reinforcement history for talking which may be correlated with the mutism.

I am unaware of a single study which has *recommended behavior changes in other people with whom the child is in contact.* We can only suppose that the increased verbal communication was reinforcing for others and that they, in turn, reinforced the verbal behavior of the previously electively mute person. Only silence which is troublesome for others receives attention and correction. Perhaps symptomatic treatment of the target problem empowers electively mute individuals to make changes in the physical setting and the behavior of others through the medium of speech and language.

Symptomatic treatment has been the almost exclusive focus of interventions for elective mutism. Except for stimulus fading there is no evidence in the elective mutism literature of changing the environment to include those factors which facilitate speaking. In the classroom, for example, a special "magic talking corner" might be useful in encouraging speaking in electively mute children. This activity could be initiated at home as suggested by Friedman and Karagan (1973) in their discussion of systematic informal treatments and later included in the target setting. The physical "props" may be gradually changed so that the setting is returned to the original physical features associated with the speech refusal.

CLASS PLACEMENT

Kehle *et al.* (1990) report that a change in placement was not successful in getting their six-year-old patient to talk. It is common for peers to accept their electively mute classmate and to offer excuses for the nonverbal behavior as well as to intercede on his or her behalf. This observation has led school personnel to place the electively mute children in a class where their problem is not known to their new classmates. The rationale for a change in class placement is that the child will talk in his new class placement because his classmates do not know him well enough to intercede on his behalf.

CHAPTER 18

BEHAVIOR MANAGEMENT PROCEDURES
PART 1

MATCHING BEHAVIOR MANAGEMENT PROCEDURES WITH ELECTIVE MUTISM CHARACTERISTICS

Williamson *et al.* (1977) offered guidelines for selecting behavior management procedures. They suggested that the first step is to identify the environmental conditions in which the child will speak. These researchers provided guidelines for identifying when to use a number of behavioral interventions.

Table 18.1. Selecting behavior management procedures.

Methods		
Contingency management*	Stimulus fading	Shaping, avoidance and escape procedures, reinforcer sampling
Low frequency speech to majority of people in target setting	Low frequency speech with one or two people in target environment	Zero speech in target setting

* Social psychologists such as Lepper and Gilovich (1981) claim that reinforcement can have an incentive function, a feedback function and a social control function. According to Lachenmeyer and Gibbs (1985), it is the second of these that allows one to evaluate the performance of electively mute persons.

Contingency management is recommended for children who are speaking at a low frequency to the majority of people in a target setting. This description of speech refusal corresponds to reluctant speech (e.g., speaking when asked a question). Stimulus fading is recommended in order to bring the child's verbal behavior under the stimulus control of new people if a child speaks to only a few people in the target environment. If the child does not talk to anyone in the target environment the therapist can either shape the child's verbal behavior, employ an avoidance procedure, use reinforcer sampling, or utilize an escape/positive reinforcement technique (Williamson *et al.*, 1977).

Many treatments for elective mutism, however, use a combination of interventions. Lazarus (1976) has used the term multimodal therapy and Knill (1978) has used the term intermodal therapy to refer to the simultaneous application of different interventions to the same person.

NON-PROFESSIONALS AS THERAPEUTIC AGENTS

Lesser-Katz (1988) suggested that the use of cotherapists is desirable in treating electively mute persons. Lesser-Katz recommended that the grandparents, teachers and peers be enlisted as cotherapists because (1) these persons are less burdened by the routine of dealing with the electively mute child and (2) cotherapy has the advantage of promoting interaction with peers and teachers. The client in the Lesser-Katz (1988) report was seen in therapy with a classroom peer with whom he was familiar. The specific role of the peer is not mentioned. But, in any event, the peer did not seem to play an active role. Instead, his presence may have reduced the anxiety of the child and, if the child talked spontaneously in the presence of the peer, the peer could have increased the likelihood of the child's beginning to talk in the new setting. Expressed technically, the presence of the peer may have functioned as a discriminative stimulus for emitting verbalizations. I have included a detailed description of peer-facilitated therapy because there seems to be ample opportunity to use peer counselors when the setting for the speech refusal is the classroom. Note[18.1] will be useful for practitioners and researchers who wish to develop peer-facilitated interventions.

PEER COUNSELING

Note[18.1]

The majority of the peer counselling programs are based on behavior therapy principles. According to Sloop (1975) the training of peer counsellors involves five processes: (1) having the students learn the principles of behavior therapy; (2) training peer-helpers to observe, and record target behaviors; (3) modeling of peer-helper tasks in the behavior change program; (4) having the peer-counsellor practice his or her role in the intervention; and (5) providing supervised practice and feedback.

Kerr and Strain (1979) offer guidelines for using peers to improve social skills of withdrawn children. These guidelines, however, are useful as general considerations for selecting peer-change agents to work with electively mute children and adolescents.
- Select a student who attends school regularly in order to promote continuity of the intervention.
- Select a student who is observed spontaneously interacting with elective mutes in a positive manner.

- Select a student who exhibits positive regard for the electively mute person.
- Select a student who can follow a teacher's verbal instructions reliably and who can imitate a teacher model.
- Select a student who is prepared to reinforce only verbalizations or responses involved in speaking, such as mouth movements.

Furthermore, learning about operant principles and the ways that social consequences affect behavior may promote self-initiated changes in the way peers interact with the individual displaying the silence user behavior.

The literature generally supports the positive way in which children and adolescents relate to their electively mute peers. It may be, therefore, advantageous to consider the option of involving peers in the treatment of electively mute peers. There are several advantages of employing peer helpers to work with electively mute persons: (1) the opportunity to work with a peer counsellor may be perceived as a positive reinforcer by the clients; (2) the opportunity to serve as a peer behavior-change agent can be a reinforcer for the person who volunteers to work with an electively mute peer; (3) in addition to getting the electively mute person to speak there may be positive side effects such as improved social relationships; (4) the peer helper may facilitate the maintenance and transfer of the client's speaking to new settings; and (5) peer counsellors permit individualized treatment of electively mute individuals.

Gartner *et al.* (1971) in *Children Teach Children: Learning by Teaching* discuss using peers as therapeutic agents. The book focuses primarily on helping students to learn academic skills by using peer tutors but a number of the guidelines apply to other contexts in which behavior change is the desired goal. Gartner *et al.* identify the characteristics of children and adolescents who will benefit from cross-age peer counselling. These include:

- Individuals who find it difficult to be successful with their own age groups.
- Children or adolescents who are the youngest in their families and who never had a chance to develop the skills of being "an older helper."
- Siblings who have not had an opportunity before to be in the same educational environment as "equals."
- A child or adolescent who has never had a chance for the close companionship of an older child.

Gartner *et al.* (1971) claim that there are several potential problems in using peers as behavior change agents. According to these authors, the problems which might be anticipated include: (1) the unrealistic expectations of a client's capabilities; (2) the tendency to do the work for the learner rather than assisting him to do it himself; (3) the tendency to be impatient and overly strict; (4) the difficulty in working with restless learners or problem children.

The following questions for assessing the effectiveness of peer counsellors appeared in the Peer Facilitator Quarterly: (1) "Did you find your meeting with this helper to be of value? If yes, how? If no, how could it have been more helpful?; (2) What did you expect in your meeting with the peer helper?; (3) Would you like to continue the relationship?; and (4) What changes have occurred as a result of your meetings?" (Gordon, 1983).

CHAPTER 19

BEHAVIOR MANAGEMENT PROCEDURES
PART 2

INTRODUCTION

Norman and Broman (1970) used a volume meter on a tape recorder to induce a child to speak, and to increase speech volume. In their intervention, speaking was reinforced only when it was loud enough to move the meter's needle into the red (loud) zone. Nolan and Pence (1970) consulted with a parent of an electively mute child and instructed the parent to gradually raise the volume of the car radio, thereby forcing the child to vocalize louder in order to be heard. Increasing the audibility of speech was also a major focus in the recent intervention reported by Brown and Doll (1988).

BROWN AND DOLL: BIOFEEDBACK PROCEDURE

In order to increase the audibility of speech the requested level of voice was demonstrated to the client in two ways (Brown and Doll, 1988). First, another child was asked to speak in an audible voice. Second, the client was asked to model the student until similarly audible speech was emitted. If the client's response to a question was audible, a "+" was recorded on the data sheet and the next question was presented. If her first response was inaudible, an "O" was recorded and she was verbally prompted to repeat her answer until it was audible. The audibility of repeated responses was not recorded.

Token Reinforcement

The client was given a card with the message, "I talked this many times" written on it. If her first response to a question was audible, the card was punched. If she received any punches the child received verbal praise from her parents and if she received a specified number of punches, she was rewarded with a vanilla milkshake by her mother.

Volume Control

During the last phase, a Voicelite[R] was placed in close proximity of the client, and she was asked to speak loudly enough to illuminate it. The Voicelite[R] is activated in response to sufficiently loud sounds and the light can be set to be illuminated at various decibel levels.

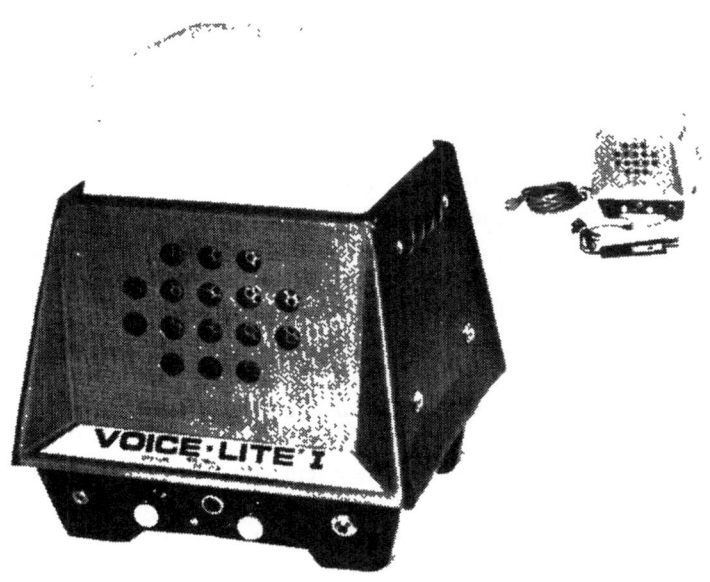

Note: For information about the Voicelite write Behavioral Controls Inc., 3818 West Mitchell Street, Milwaukee, WI 53215, USA or fax 1–414–671–3332. Reproduced with permission of Behavioral Controls, Inc.

Fig. 19.1. Voicelite[R] used in the Brown and Doll procedure.

In the Brown and Doll (1988) intervention, Voicelite[R] was set at approximately 20 decibels, the volume of the typical speaking voice. The client continued to be verbally prompted to speak louder and to take home a punch card of the number of verbal responses she had made which illuminated the Voicelite[R] on the first trial.

Withdrawal Phase

The withdrawal procedure used by Brown and Doll (1988) continued to use the Voicelite^R but the verbal prompts for louder speech were discontinued as was the use of punch cards. There was little or no change, however, in the frequency of loud responses but there was an increase in the frequency of episodes of whispered speech.

NORMAN AND BROMAN: BIOFEEDBACK PROCEDURE

Norman and Broman (1970) described a successful treatment of a 12-year-old boy using shaping by volume control and visual feedback. The treatment progressed through several phases: (a) reinforcing sounds and noises with a soft drink, (b) increasing volume of client's sounds and noises with visual feedback from the volume meter on a tape recorder, (c) responding to questions with one word responses rather than noises, (d) naming objects and briefly describing events in slides, and (e) talking in the presence of classmates, the school counsellor, other teachers, and principal.

Reinforcement of Vocal Sounds

The first phase established rapport with the client and acquainted the child with the treatment plan. At this point, the client refused to open his mouth and it was necessary to verbally prompt him into making sounds. This was done by the therapist making "funny faces." In each instance, the client was observed to smile and emit a low volume noise. Every time the client made a noise he was positively reinforced with a sip of soft drink. Next, a verbal request for sound was introduced and sounds were reinforced with a sip of soft drink. After receiving reinforcement for making sounds, the child was asked to make a sound while his lips were parted. The child did as requested and was again reinforced with a sip of drink. Requests for louder sounds, however, were unsuccessful during this phase.

Increasing the Volume of Vocal Sounds

A tape recorder was introduced to raise the volume of sounds emitted by the child as well as to shape speech sounds. The volume meter permitted the client to receive one of three forms of visual feedback after each request to make louder sounds: (1) the child did not respond and the needle did not move; (2) the child responded softly and the needle moved into the gray;

(3) the child responded loudly and the needle moved into the black. See Fig. 19.2.

Initially, the volume meter was set at its most sensitive audio level and the child was asked to make sounds. This setting meant that the child's voice had to be barely audible to move the needle into the black area of the volume meter. No response or the needle moving into the gray was followed by the therapist saying "louder." Next, the therapist adjusted the volume control so that the child had to make progressively louder sounds in order to move the needle into the black area. After every five reinforced trials, the volume of the recorder was lowered a half step.

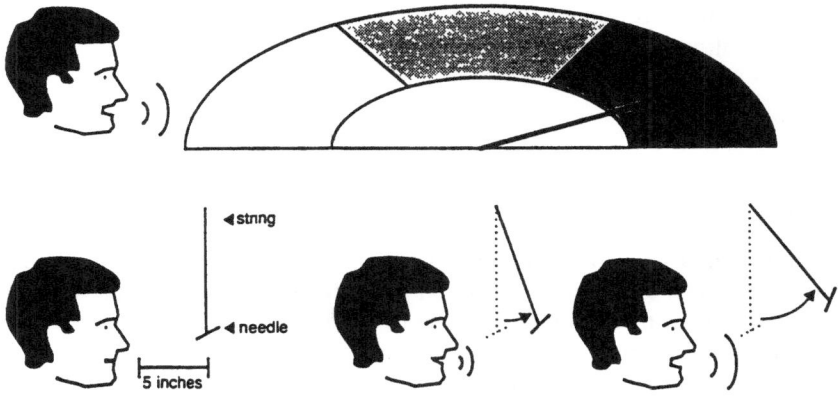

The figure illustrates the type of visual feedback described by Norman and Broman (1970). In this example, the client's voice was loud enough to activate the volume meter and to move the needle into the black area of the scale. According to the Norman and Broman (1970) guidelines, a verbalization of this volume qualified the speaker for reinforcement. The bottom section of the Figure illustrates how a string with a needle attached to it can be used to provide visual feedback for speaking (Lipton, 1970).

Fig. 19.2. Volume meter of tape recorder employed as biofeedback instrument and string with needle attached biofeedback method.

Shaping Responses

During this phase, the child was asked to shape his sounds into words, with food as the reinforcer. The child was told to say "ugh" if he wanted food and "ugg, ugg" if he did not. An affirmative response was shaped into "yuh," then into "yeh" and finally "yes." The sounds for "no" were shaped into "uh, uh" and later the client modelled the word "no." After the child attained a stable pattern of responding with "yes" and "no," he was urged to name objects in the room and to read simple sentences. The child received tokens for correct responses, which later could be exchanged for food. The use of tokens introduced a delay between making the required response and receiving reinforcement, thereby preventing the child from becoming satiated on food reinforcers.

Responding to Events in Slides

During this phase of the Norman and Broman (1970) procedure the focus was on getting the child to talk to individuals to whom he would be expected to talk in the school setting. Reinforced by tokens, the child was asked to name people and objects depicted in slides and later to respond to the slides with short phrases and sentences.

Speech Generalization

The tape recorder was again used during the last phase. The volume meter was adjusted so that a low volume of sound moved the needle. After the client responded with low volume responses, the meter was set at the level of normal speech and the use of token reinforcement was reinstated. This adjustment meant that a louder volume of speech was required in order to move the needle into the black area of the volume meter scale.

Stimulus fading was conducted in the therapist's office. The door was closed and the child was told that there was a person behind the door and that he could see more of the person if he said "hello." The boy was asked to say "hello" and if he did not respond he was verbally prompted by the therapist. After emitting several "hellos" with the door closed, it was opened slightly but the stranger was not visible. The next set of "hellos" made the person partially visible, and each successive five "hellos" increased the visibility of the stranger until the entire person was visible. Continued speaking by the child brought the person closer and eventually into the room. At this point, social reinforcement in the form of praise and smiles were dispensed by both the therapist and the stranger. At the end of this phase, Norman and Broman (1970) reported that the child's responses to the therapist's questions increased by 50% and his responses to the new person's questions increased by 37%.

ALBERT-STEWART: BIOFEEDBACK PROCEDURE

Albert-Stewart (1986) reported that her electively mute client used short sentences and spoke in a monotone. Much of what the boy said could not be heard because he spoke in a whisper. When the author instructed him to speak audibly, he responded with periodic bursts of elevated volume but his speech was not consistently audible or intelligible. When confronted with these observations the child claimed that he was speaking loudly enough to be heard and clearly enough to be understood. Albert-Stewart indicated that the discovery of the client's misconception influenced her to use a treatment based on positive reinforcement and biofeedback. The author collaborated with the client in designing the treatment which consisted of immediate praise, contingent awarding of points, and exchanging points for a prize when he earned a predetermined number of points.

The biofeedback component of the treatment consisted of the following sequence of events. First, the client was asked to read from fiction books into the microphone connected to a tape recorder, and to speak loudly enough to keep a red volume light continuously illuminated while he was reading. Each time the task was performed correctly, he earned immediate praise from the therapist. Inaudible speech was ignored. The second phase of the intervention involved placing the tape recorder 5 feet away from the client while he read. The tape recorder was positioned 10 feet away when the client met the criterion for audible speech at a distance of 5 feet. When he spoke loudly enough to activate the volume light at 10 feet, the tape recorder was returned to the desk in front of him. Albert-Stewart (1986) reported that although the client improved in raising the volume of his voice, he continued to speak unintelligibly when he encountered unfamiliar words.

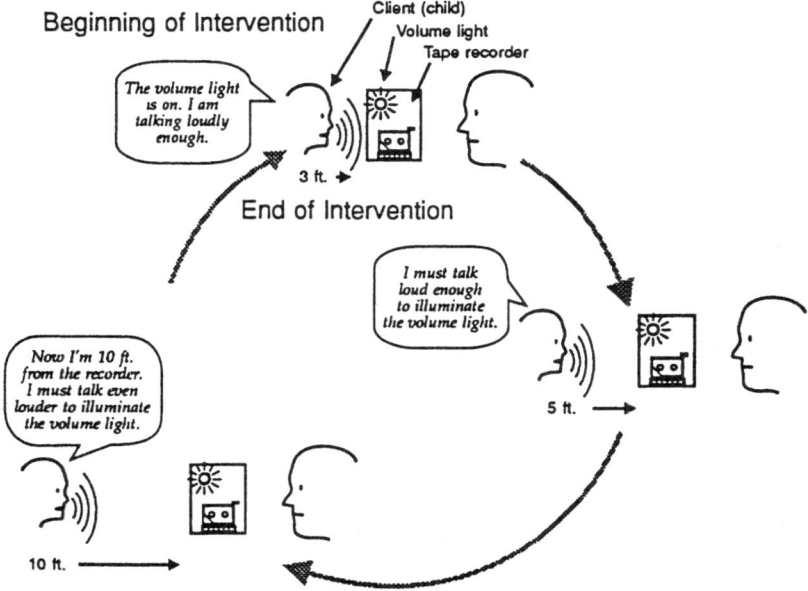

Fig. 19.3. Biofeedback procedure of Albert-Stewart.

LISTENING TO THE EVOLVING THERAPEUTIC RELATIONSHIP

The administration of positive stimuli may not necessarily have a reinforcing effect on the response of speaking. Observation, however, may reveal that behaviors connected with building a relationship are strengthened. For example, Shreeve (1991) observed that when he praised his four-year-old electively mute client, she drew closer but rarely made eye contact. This shows how important it is to be watchful of nonverbal behaviors. With the exception of motoric behavior, inner responses such as affect and imagery cannot be directly observed but depend on the client's self-report. The self-report of electively mute persons need not take the form of verbal behavior. For example, a feeling, image, or thought may be expressed in a drawing, sculpture, or in a "mime-type" response. Krolian (1988), for example, monitored vocal behavior such as laughing and, like other researchers, observed low volume utterances (whispering) prior to their speaking in a conversational voice.

Krolian (1988) emphasized that mutism should not be the initial target for intervention because such an initial target will only increase the silence and oppositional behavior. He claimed that nonverbal expressions should be considered communications worthy of exploration and interpretation. Krolian (1988), therefore, prioritized getting to know the client. He believed that this could be achieved by "listening" to the client's nonverbal responses.

BEHAVIORAL DESENSITIZATION TREATMENT

Note[19.1]

Desensitization therapy is a form of psychotherapy in which a patient learns to extinguish unwanted emotional responses to certain stimuli. This is accomplished through a process of repeated exposure to these stimuli either in real life or fantasy.

Fear management involves exposing the client to gradually increasing intensities of the fear stimulus. In the case of elective mutism, this means encouraging the client to speak in a setting in which he elects not to speak. As illustrated in the schematic, there are several ways of exposing the electively mute person to the fear stimulus.

One way of exposing a client to a fear stimulus is to begin at the bottom of the ladder which corresponds to the least fear arousing stimulus. Since the client does not talk, the hierarchy of fear stimuli must be based on the therapist's observations of the client in speaking and non-speaking environments and information from the child's parents, peers and teachers.

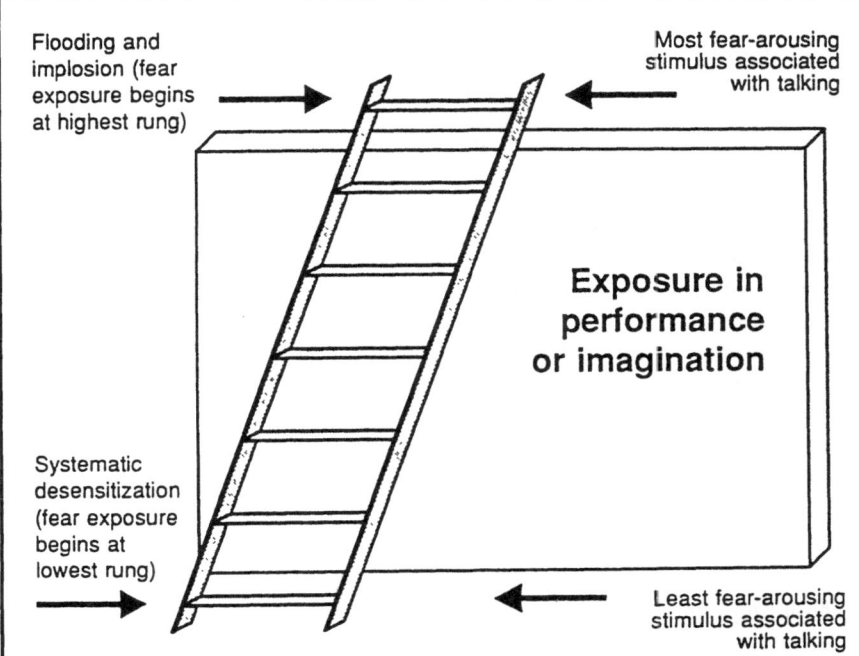

Flooding and implosion (fear exposure begins at highest rung)

Most fear-arousing stimulus associated with talking

Exposure in performance or imagination

Systematic desensitization (fear exposure begins at lowest rung)

Least fear-arousing stimulus associated with talking

Exposure

Systematic exposure can be achieved in two ways: (1) in imagination by having the client "picture" himself on the lowest rung (for elective mutism, to imagine the least fearful communication such as playing a game with the therapist which does not require speaking) and (2) in vivo exposure by having the client "actually stand on the lowest rung of the ladder." In treating elective mutism this could correspond to having the client actually play a game without talking to the therapist in a setting in which the client elects to speak. Positive reinforcement is administered when a client indicates that she has imagined the first step or actually "stands on the first rung." With elective mutism, exposure in imagination would not be recommended because the client would not be expected to verbalize the details of her image and her reactions to the image. The therapist would have no way of monitoring the client's imagery or even of knowing if the client's imagery was focused on the target problem. The overt performance of the client during in vivo exposure, however, permits the therapist to monitor the client's progress as well as to observe the nonverbal responses (e.g., facial expression and trembling) which accompany the approach behavior. The client should remain on each successive rung of the ladder until there is evidence that the fear has subsided.

Cautions in Using Exposure

If in vivo exposure is used it is important to consider the consequences of permitting the client to step down from the ladder before the fear has subsided. If the client leaves the ladder before the fear is reduced, he may inadvertently reinforce himself through the relief which accompanies the escape from the fear stimulus. Therefore, the client should be positively reinforced for staying on the ladder. This raises another important issue. When using in vivo exposure, it is recommended that a therapy session be ended when the client exhibits minimal fear. Ending a session when the client is fearful permits the client to escape the fear situation and this could reinforce the fear response.

Modeling and Exposure

Modeling can also be used with in vivo exposure. The therapist can demonstrate what he wishes the client to do (e.g., speaking softly into a tape recorder and playing back the recorded message). Modeling also has important implications for treatment. Research indicates that a coping model is more effective than a mastery model. A model which exhibits some fear together with coping responses for dealing with the fear is more effective than a fearless model. A coping model for overcoming fear of heights could include statements such as "Well, this task will not be easy, but I can do it. I shall just take my time. I shall step slowly on the first rung of the ladder and make sure my feet are securely placed. I will hold onto the rungs." In contrast, a mastery or fearless model is reflected in statements such as "Watch me, it's easy" (followed by the therapist's climbing quickly to the top). "See, nothing happened. Come on up." Not only would the client have difficulty in identifying with the fearless behavior, but in addition a fearless model does not include guidelines for coping with the fear. A coping model for getting a client to talk in a target environment might include statements such as "Watch me, I know this is not going to be easy, but I know I can do it. I am going to turn on the tape recorder. I shall slowly and softly say the three words printed on the card – one at a time, slowly and in a soft voice." Electively mute individuals would be likely to identify with the coping model and, in addition, they would have a practical model to follow for speaking in the fearful situation.

Flooding

The therapist could also place the client at the top rung of the ladder. This fear management method of initially exposing the client to the highest intensity of the fear stimulus is called flooding. The client is exposed to the greatest fear stimulus in the hierarchy. Flooding, like systematic desensitization, can be done through in vivo exposure or in imagination. It is possible that flooding could inadvertently occur even in systematic desensitization because it may not be possible to break down the fear into small enough gradations so that the fear is minimally experienced by the client. If fear is increased during exposure, systematic desensitization corresponds to high intensity exposure to the fear stimulus, and the therapist should proceed with flooding while keeping in mind the guideline of not letting the client leave the ladder until the fear subsides.

Exposure in Person-Centred Therapy

In person-centred therapy the client generates his own fear hierarchy and gradually exposes himself to the fear. When the clients begin therapy, they make disclosures involving minimal anxiety and, as therapy progresses, their disclosures typically include progressively more anxiety-arousing material. In person-centred therapy, exposure takes the form of revealing and discussing in the presence of the therapist the components of the client's self-generated fear hierarchy and subjective reactions to them. The client may also assign herself "homework." What seems to occur in person-centred treatment of fears is that the client approaches the fear situation in words and later in action outside of therapy (Martin, 1972). The client also develops insight into her self-defeating images and cognitions. The client must *talk about* the images, affects, sensations, and cognitions which contribute to her elective mutism. Therefore, symptomatic treatment (getting the child to talk) must precede insight therapy. The exception seems to be the expressive therapies in which insight may develop simultaneously with or even before talking occurs.

FADING TREATMENT OF ELECTIVE MUTISM

With respect to the treatment of elective mutism, stimulus fading refers to one of two procedures. Fading involves, first, gradually introducing characteristics of the setting in which the child elects to be silent or, second, gradually removing characteristics of the setting in which the child elects to talk so that the setting comes closer and closer to the one in which the client elects not to talk. In either case, conversational speech gradually occurs to stimuli which have been associated with not speaking. In stimulus fading, the client is often asked to read while the distance between the client and a parent is increased, and the distance between the client and a teacher or stranger is decreased. According to Sanok and Ascione (1979) and Cunningham *et al.* (1983), stimulus fading coupled with reinforcement is currently the most effective treatment for elective mutism.

Wassing: Fading Procedure

Wassing (1973) described how a tape recorder was used in a systematic in vivo desensitization procedure. The first phase involved establishing a relationship with the client by using a game which did not require verbal participation. During this activity the therapist explained the treatment to the client. In *Phase 2*, the client was asked to read aloud in the absence of the therapist. While they listened to the client's tape, the client received encouraging comments from the therapist. During *Phase 3*, the client was required to read aloud into the microphone in the presence of the therapist. In order to minimize nonverbal evaluative responses, the therapist read a book with his back turned to the client. *Phase 4* differs from the preceding one because the therapist faced the client from a position diagonally opposite him at a distance of two meters. When the client began to speak into the tape recorder, the therapist did not look at the client but resumed "reading."

During *Phase 5*, the therapist continued to "read" while the client was talking but he shortened the distance to one meter and changed his position so that he was sitting directly in front of the client. In *Phase 6* the therapist attentively listened to the client's reading aloud. The therapist not only stopped "reading" but occasionally looked at the client while he was reading. At the conclusion of Phase 6, the client was reading aloud in the presence of the therapist. During *Phase 7*, the client wrote his answers to the therapist's questions and read them to the therapist. *Phase 8* was similar to the previous phase except that the client replied to the therapist's questions without referring to his written answers. *Phase 9* involved a major transition. The client began answering questions in phrases or sentences without using notes. With the removal of the mutistic response, the final phase marked the transition from symptomatic to insight therapy. The insight phase is not discussed by Wassing.

Conrad, Delk and Williams: Fading Procedure

The Conrad *et al.* (1974) treatment of a six-year-old electively mute girl began with symptomatic treatment and concluded with insight therapy. *Phase 1* was conducted in the client's home with the mother and therapist present. The mother asked the child to respond to the therapist's questions. Simple arithmetic problems on flashcards served as questions and responses were reinforced with candy on a continuous reinforcement schedule.

Phases 2 and 3 were also conducted in the home but the mother was not present and a 10:1 fixed ratio reinforcement schedule was used. The fourth and fifth phases were conducted in a clinic setting in the absence of the mother. A friend of the child participated in order to make the treatment setting more like the classroom. Flashcards were again used and the client and peer were asked to use the words in sentences, but only complete sentences reinforced.

Phases 6–9 were clinic-based and the therapist, peer and the teacher were present. The teacher presented the flash cards. Reinforcement in the form of points which could be exchanged for tangible reinforcers was administered on a fixed ratio schedule of 10:1. The setting for *Phase 10* was the classroom. Present were the client, the therapist, the teacher, and five classmates selected by the teacher. Flash cards continued to serve as stimuli for verbal responses. Questions were directed to individual children with the client being asked to respond to one out of every six questions. Responses to questions were reinforced on a fixed-ratio schedule of 10:1. The final two phases were identical to *Phase 10* except that the class was present. A follow-up at one year revealed that the child continued to respond verbally to the teacher when directly spoken to but rarely initiated conversations with her.

Reid, Hawkins, Keutzer, McNeal, Phelps, Reid and Mees: Fading Procedure

Reid *et al.* (1973) described a three-phase fading technique based on the observation that elective mutism was related to a fear of strangers. In *Phase 1*, the therapist established a constant rate of speaking between the mother and child by having the child ask the mother for food. In the training procedure, the mother asked the client if she wanted a bite of food at 30 second intervals. A verbal request for food, including its identification (e.g., "orange juice" to "I'd like some banana, please, Mummie"), was required in order to receive it. If no response occurred, the mother waited for 30 seconds and tried again.

The second phase of the treatment involved fading a stranger into the playroom while the client continued to request food from her mother. The stranger moved from a location in the hall to one of the chairs at the table in steps of approximately three feet. There were 10 positions through which the stranger moved while pretending to read a magazine. The criterion for the stranger to move to each closer position was several consecutive verbal responses from the client. The client was observed becoming more verbal as the stranger was faded into the room. Reid *et al.* (1973) reported that 43 verbal responses from the child were required for the stranger to move from the hall to the table. The client's verbal responses increased from an average of 1.7 words on the first 10 trials to 2.6 words on the last 10.

Phase 3 involved shaping the client to look at and respond to the stranger. This was accomplished by fading the stranger into the mother-child conversation. At regular intervals, the stranger asked the client's mother, "Why don't you ask her if she would like another bite to eat?" The mother asked the questions and the client responded. After the child had responded to two of the mother's questions in the presence of the stranger, the stranger directly asked the client "Would you like something more?" From this point on, the stranger asked the client at 30 second intervals if she wanted another bite to eat. She responded but did not look at the stranger. After several trials, the stranger moved his chair directly opposite the client so that she would have to look at him while requesting food. Within 15 trials from sitting opposite the client, the stranger was carrying on a limited conversation with the child.

MULTI-MODAL TREATMENT OF ELECTIVE MUTISM

In the Schmerling and Kerins (1987) case study, there are eight phases in the treatment. The first phase emphasized teaching the child to do smooth-easy inhalations and exhalations. The specific focus was on encouraging the child to forcefully blow. *Phase 2* saw the introduction of gesturing to de-emphasize the demands for verbalizations. The use of gesturing acknowledged that speech was difficult for the child, yet provided him with a means of communicating.

The emphasis on vocal behavior in *Phase 3* developed out of breathing exercises. This was accomplished by having the child blow fruit loops across the table. As a consequence, the therapist rewarded the child with a fruit loop. Later, the game was continued, but this time the activity was made into a playful contest between the child and a peer. *Phase 4* involved the therapist's setting up a simulated classroom setting with the child and some of his peers. The child asked for objects, first, by gesturing and, later, by producing initial sounds. Responsivity was noted by observing if the client: (1) rigidly held the body immobile, (2) maintained eye contact, and (3) held his breath when in a group setting. Opening and closing rituals involved using a drum to say "hello" or "good bye" to the therapist and peers. *Phase 5* focused on encouraging social interaction by prompting the electively mute child to mouth the names of peers so they could guess to whom he was speaking. Also, an activity which approximated "Simon says" involving motoric responses such as "head-nodding" and "arm-swinging" was used. The child was in control of the responses and peers imitated his responses. In the beginning of *Phase 6*, as in the earlier phases, the therapist initiated communication. A number of activities were used which simulated parent-child games including (1) peek-a-boo, (2) hide-and-seek, and (3) hide the elbow.

GAME PLAY

Note[19.2]

I have used the term "game play" to place the technique of Schmerling and Kerins (1987) into a framework which yields generic characteristics. Because some of my readers may be less familiar with game play than they are with the psychology of play and play therapy, I thought it might be advantageous to explain how game play differs from play. Game play does differ from play yet it shares two characteristics of play – both game play and play are intended to be fun and provide an opportunity for fantasy experience. In contrast to play, however, all games have rules which set the expectations and limits for behavior. Games usually involve a contest – a defined set of rules in order to produce a winner. Indeed, Sutton-Smith and Roberts (1971) claim that games are "models for power . . . with which children and adolescents learn socially acceptable ways to succeed over others." The edited monograph by Schaefer and Reid (1986) provides an elaborated definition of game play:

- Playing a game is an enjoyable activity.
- Games have an "as if" quality that separates them from real life and allows for fantasy experience.
- Rules exist, or are created, that define and restrict the behavior of the players and add organization and structure to the game.
- A contest is implied or explicit in games, in that players compete either with each other or with themselves in order to win the game.
- Games, by virtue of their structured, competitive makeup pose a challenge to the participants. At the lowest level, the challenge is to play with other people in a self-controlled, cooperative fashion.

> More complex games require more in terms of emotional control,
> intellect, and social skills.
> • Game-playing usually involves interaction between two or more
>   players (p. 4).

Prior to introducing the option of a walkie-talkie in *Phase 7*, the clinician provided a broad range of options for making sounds such as a whistle,
a flute, and rhythm instruments. The favorite "prop" of the electively mute
child, however, was a walkie-talkie. Schmerling and Kerins (1987) believed
that this was surprising because the person using the walkie-talkie cannot
rely upon nonverbal expression or gestures. It seems possible, however, that
the advantage of using a walkie-talkie in the treatment of elective mutism
is that it permits the silence user to converse without seeing his speaking
partner. Initially, the walkie-talkie was used to blow, cough, and sneeze
into it. In *Phase 8*, the child was exposed to dance-movement activities. The
patient used the signed words and sounds that he was using during his
speech-language therapy sessions in the dance and movement activities.
Schmerling and Kerins (1987) argued that "carrying" a prop from one
session to the next was a sign that an effective bridge was being made.

CHAPTER 20

SELF-MODELING

DEFINITION

Dowrick and Dove (1980) defined self-modeling as "the behavioral change that results from the repeated observation of oneself on videotapes that show only desired target behaviors" (p. 51). The modeling tape is made and the child observes the edited videotape of himself or herself performing the desired behavior at a greater frequency than his or her present functioning.

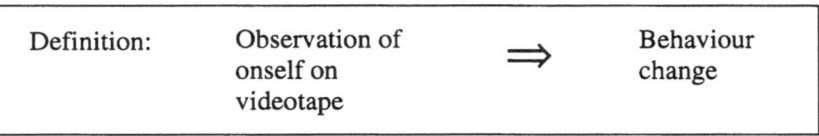

Fig. 20.1. Self-modeling.

ADVANTAGES

There are several advantages of self-modeling treatment of elective mutism. First, the method is time efficient. Parents can be enlisted as mediators to make the videotape of the child's talking and this means that the therapist's time can be spent performing a behavioral assessment and editing the videotape. Second, most children have a positive association with television, and they like seeing themselves on the television. Third, the model is the client with the problem and this enhances the modeling effect because no model could be more similar than the child himself or herself. Fourth, there is strong theoretical support that self-modeling enhances self-efficacy (Kehle *et al.*, 1990).

PROCEDURE

Pigott and Gonzales (1987) used self-modeling in an educational setting to treat a third-grade elective mute. A behavioral analysis revealed that the child would respond to questions in the presence of his mother and brother. Consequently, the researchers prepared videotapes of the client's talking in the presence of these people.

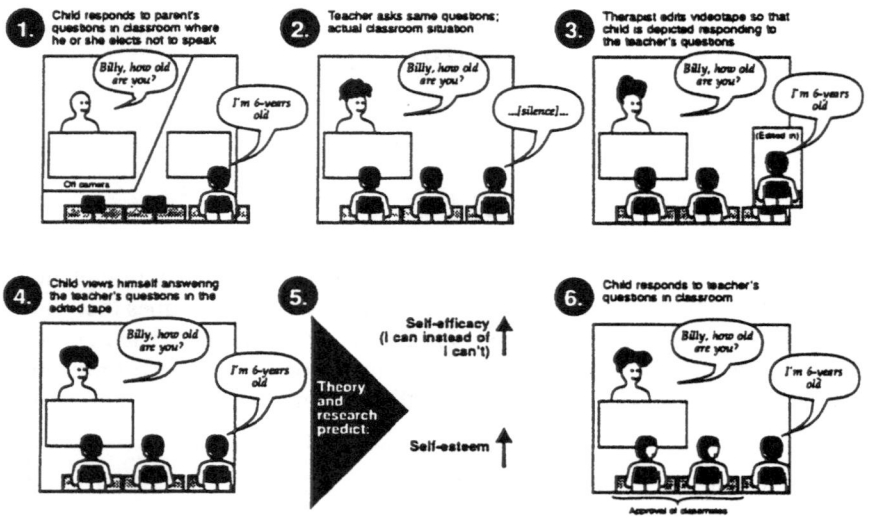

Fig. 20.2. Self-modeling treatment of elective mutism.

In positive self-modeling, two videotapes must be made. In the case of elective mutism, one videotape is made of the child answering a set of questions in the setting in which he elects to talk and a second tape is made of the child refusing to answer the same questions in a setting in which the client refuses to talk. In order to facilitate the editing of the video-tape, it is important to position the person to whom the client talks near to the child, but off-camera. Before the video is made of the setting in which the child elects not to talk, it is important to obtain signed releases which authorize the videotaping of the other children in the setting.

EDITING THE VIDEOTAPE

Editing involves "moving" the child's answers from a videotape in which the client replied to his mother's questions to the videotape in which the teacher asked him the same set of questions. In other words, the client's answers to his mother's questions (i.e., the same questions asked by the teacher) are "put in" as answers to the teacher's questions to which the client did not respond.

VIEWING INSTRUCTIONS

There seems to be no clear-cut recommendations for this activity. There are advantages, however, of having the child view the videotape in the setting in which he or she elects to be silent. But, if the child's parents or child does not agree to this, the child can view the videotape at home. Pigott and Gonzales (1987) instructed the parents to arrange for the child to observe the videotape prior to attending school.

SELF-MONITORING: TOWARD NATURAL SELF-MODELING

Self-observation and self-recording are associated with producing and maintaining behavior changes (Maletzky, 1974; McFall, 1976; Kanfer and Gaelick-Buys, 1991). But in order to use this approach the person must emit the behavior to be self-monitored and self-recorded. Hence, self-monitoring procedures are best applied after exposing the person to self-modeling.

In the Pigott and Gonzales (1987) study, the child periodically took the card on which he recorded episodes of speaking to the teacher for her to acknowledge his participation. The teacher circled the number corresponding to the self-reported speaking episodes and signed the card, and the child took the card home to inform his parents about his progress. In consultation with the author, a point-reinforcement system was instituted so that a defined number of hand-raises and responses to questions earned a backup reinforcer of the child's choosing (Pigott and Gonzales, 1987).

SEQUENCE OF TAPES

It may be necessary to make several self-modeling videotapes to help the student bridge the gap between reluctant speech and spontaneous speech. Reluctant or responsive speakers will answer questions which are directed to them, but they will not volunteer to answer questions or spontaneously elaborate on questions which are directed to them. The clinician should first make a self-modeling tape for answering questions. This tape is intended to move the child from an electively mute phase to an intermediate phase between silence user and spontaneous speech. The videotape which bridges this gap shows the child answering questions which are directed to him or her. A subsequent self-modeling videotape would depict the client initiating speech and elaborating on his or her responses.

CHARTING SPEAKING EPISODES

There is an advantage of charting the child's progress. The graph provides visual feedback and this may reinforce the child's speaking in class. The change in the target behavior is also a potent reinforcer for the mediator who is working directly with the child (Tharp and Wetzel, 1969). The visual inspection of the data also permits assessment of the internal validity of the intervention. Determining if an intervention is responsible for the behavior change is termed internal validity.

CHAPTER 21

EXPRESSIVE THERAPY INTERVENTIONS
PART 1

CHARACTERISTICS

Expressive therapy refers to the therapeutic application of the creative arts to human problems. Expressive therapy uses the "power of the arts experience to improve the quality of human lives and thereby expand human horizons" (Warren, 1984, p. vii). Art therapy, dance and movement therapy, music therapy, phototherapy and poetry therapy are expressive therapies. Furthermore, pet-facilitated therapy, play therapy, sand tray therapy, and game play therapy also readily fit into the philosophy and framework of the expressive therapies. This chapter will not make the reader an expressive therapist nor will it provide a pancrea for the problem of elective mutism. However, it will give insight into some of the approaches originating in the expressive therapies that have been beneficial in treating persons who elect to be silence users.

There are few published reports that I know of which use dance-movement therapy, drama therapy, and fairytale-facilitated therapy in treating elective mutism. Expressive therapy treatments of elective mutism are limited to the modalities of art and play. These expressive therapies would be useful in combination with symptomatic treatment because the electively mute client, at least initially, does not use verbal behavior to communicate during therapy. As professionals in the mental health field become more aware of the expressive therapies, we shall probably see more published reports of treatments based on dance, drama, music and art. This chapter primarily reviews the role of the modalities of art and play in treating elective mutism.

WORKING ALONGSIDE THE CLIENT

A review of the art therapy literature indicates two contrasting stances on the therapists' working on their own art while the clients work on their art. The positive view is represented in the works of Haeseler (1987) and Lachman-Chapin (1983) while the opposing view is represented by Wadeson (1986).

Positive Stance

The therapist's attending to her own art work provides privacy for the client and seems to put many clients at ease (Haeseler, 1987). Supportive of this position is the interactive technique of Lachman-Chapin (1983) which aims to assist clients to discuss their own and others' art work. In this approach, the client makes a picture and the therapist makes a picture in response to the drawing. The client then feels understood and validated. The client, seeing the personal investment of the therapist in the art work, will consider his own involvement meaningful (Haeseler, 1986).

Haeseler (1986) also stresses that the clinicians working on their own art alongside the patients helps to reduce the intensity of the client-therapist relationship. Through art, the therapist and patient can exchange "thoughts" without anyone "losing face" because the focus of the interactions is on the art work rather than on each other. If therapists produce art alongside their clients, this allows them to get to know their clients and, in turn, this process hastens the development of the therapeutic relationship. While therapists and clients are creating their own art products, the clients are given the opportunity to observe and model some of the therapists' behavior. This approach gives clients an opportunity to try out the therapists style of working or to borrow their images and make them their own.

Opposing Position

In contrast to the above position Wadeson (1986) does not favor therapists producing their own art work while they are working with their clients. She cites four reasons in support of this position: (1) the therapeutic focus is the client's problems, not the therapist's; (2) for clients who feel inadequate in art, the more experienced drawings of the therapist might be intimidating; (3) the processing of the therapist's art work consumes valuable therapy time which could be more profitably spent in exploring the patient's art productions; and (4) the therapist might become so involved in her own art expression that she might inadvertently neglect the client.

Discussion

In spite of Wadeson's counter position, I would suggest that it is especially important for the art therapist to work alongside the electively mute person. The fact that such clients rarely talk to their therapists early in treatment makes verbal behavior unsuitable. Making art with the electively mute client helps the client to share his art with the therapist and lessens the threat of communicating verbally. As the client becomes more relaxed in image-making and sharing, I would recommend reducing the amount of time the art therapist spends on his or her own art work in order to give priority to the client and his or her art work.

EARLY BRITISH CONTRIBUTION

Salfield: Expressive Therapies

Salfield (1950) reported about a seven-year-old mute boy who was referred for treatment because he never spoke to his teacher. At the time of referral he refused to use pencil or chalk. Occasionally, he wrote numbers in his exercise book but not those that he was asked to copy from the black-board. He compressed his lips when speech was expected.

After about six months, William could be coaxed into answering questions in monosyllables, but he replied only when the answer was suggested. The other children were instructed to encourage the child to participate in their play. This led to his speaking to other children in whispers. When no further progress seemed likely, the psychologist treated William and one other child together. It appears that the second child was not electively mute. The process was reported as follows:

The psychologist played some game with this one child. William was free to take part in the game, and was always invited and given his turn to play, but the game went on whether William joined in or not (p. 1026).

Although the psychologist attempted to interest William in play activities, he refused to touch the play materials during the first month of treatment. After the first month, however, he began to reach for play materials and to play with them. Furthermore, he produced two drawings, one of a tractor and one of a road roller going toward a little boy whom he identified as his baby brother. At this point, Salfield reported that the child spontaneously described the two drawings. The two drawings in combination were interpreted as "sibling rivalry." However, aside from an intuitive data base, reasons for this interpretation were not identified. Salfield also said that the boy often produced scribbles, but the implications of these for treatment were not discussed. On another occasion, he said that the child drew what vaguely resembled a truck. The author said that:

. . . when he was praised for it, and asked what it was, his reply was misinterpreted as "lorry" but he was told it did not quite look like one, and a lorry was drawn for him as a model. He became angry and said "You are daft," and went on in this vein for some time, and finally it came out that what he had drawn was a tractor (p. 1026).

At the conclusion of therapy, Salfield indicated that William was observed to spontaneously join the other children in play and although he began to speak freely to relatives and strangers at home he continued to be mute at school.

Discussion

The patient freely produced two drawings and spontaneously described these drawings. Other than a statement about the client's reaction to the therapist's calling his "tractor" a "lorry" little else is said about his drawings. The observation that he produced scribbles is not elaborated upon; nor is the significance of this behavior indicated. Although client-produced drawings and scribbles are mentioned in the treatment section of the article, there is little evidence that the process of drawing was systematically used to obtain information about the target response. Furthermore, drawing and scribbling appeared to have no function other than providing a context for talking. In defense of the approach, however, it is safe to say that the patient found it easier to talk about his drawings than he did to talk about himself. Because a number of approaches were applied at approximately the same time it is impossible to attribute the behavior change to the art therapy procedures which were employed.

EARLY AMERICAN STUDIES

Parker, Olsen and Throckmorton

Part I: Play Therapy

Parker *et al.* (1960) identified nonverbal behaviors which the clinician could observe during assessment and treatment. These observations could be viewed as a continuum of involvement ranging from the patient's observing the physical setting, touching but not playing with toys or art materials, picking up toys or art materials to examine them, and playing with toys and using art materials. Schematically this might be represented as follows:

Sitting/standing/observing		Picking up/manipulating/ toys/art materials	
↓	2	↓	4
1	↓	3	↑
	Touching toys/ art materials		Playing with toys/ using art materials

Fig. 21.1. Continuum showing progressive involvement with play materials.

Because the patient does not speak, it is helpful if the clinician attempts to verbalize the actions of the patient (e.g., "I am standing in the doorway looking at the toys"). The therapist may wish to go beyond reflecting on what the client is doing, however, to include hypotheses about what the patient might be thinking and feeling. In addition to intuition, statements about cognitions and affect should be based on careful observations of the nonverbal expressions of the electively mute persons. Parker *et al.* (1960) illustrate this sequence in their case study of Deena:

> The first session Deena stood the whole time, but in the second hour after about twenty minutes she touched some of the toys in a gingerly way but did not play with them. In the third session she picked up some of the dolls and put them back in the box. During this time she was telling the mother that she liked to come to see me because there were so many things to play with. By the fourth session Deena manipulated the toys as soon as she came into the room, moving some of the toy cars one after another (p. 69).

It may be advantageous to extend the right side of the continuum so that it could be used for summarizing patient progress after the initial phases of treatment. Sample items for additional points on the scale include: (1) covering the mouth with the hand while speaking; (2) giggling aloud; and (3) speaking when the therapist turns his back to the patient or when the patient turns his back to the therapist, perhaps communicating, "I find it easier to talk if we are not looking at each other."

Parker *et al.* (1960) discussed the guidelines for interviewing parents of electively mute children. According to these writers, information that the child does not talk at school when he does talk at home may come as a surprise to the parents. The authors indicate, however, that more often than not the parents are very aware of their child's shyness with strangers, including other children. In spite of this, the parents may feel that the school in some way contributed to the problem.

The parents, therefore, need the sensitive understanding of the therapist as they try to understand their child's problem and their own bewilderment. According to Parker *et al.* (1960):

> The task of remembering occurrences, dates, and sequences uses the parent's concern in a constructive manner and allays the possible threat of their inadequacy in the parental role (p. 68).

Although Parker *et al.* (1960) were not operating within a behavioral framework, I believe that the interview focus closely parallels behavioral interviewing – especially the more traditional form in which "Where?," "When?," "How?," and "Who?" questions are favored over opinion or etiological "Why?" questions.

Part II: Expressions in Clay

The "let's pretend" approach (Parker *et al.*, 1960) was used to encourage an electively mute child to express himself through the medium of clay. This approach was also intended to allay anxiety. Parker *et al.* (1960) describe how the technique was used with a child who had briefly experienced dental trauma and separation from the mother while the dentist was treating the child. The trauma occurred when the patient was having two abscessed teeth removed and after the dentist had sent the mother out of the room. The researchers underscore the observation that the trauma occurred while the child was *beginning to speak*. I contend that the procedure of extracting the teeth *undoubtedly prevented him from speaking during the peak moments of pain and anxiety*. The authors argued that the mouth trauma involved pain and anxiety, and this influenced the choice of symptom which was expressed in later anxiety-arousing circumstances. Parker *et al.* (1960) described the sequence during structured sculpturing activities with their three-and-a-half year old electively mute child:

> I moved on to the use of clay. With the comment that I had to go to the dentist to get my teeth fixed, I made a shallow bowl of clay which, with bits of clay affixed to the rims for teeth, might pass for the mouth cavity. Martin copied my activity. In response to my comment that I hoped the dentist would not hurt me, Martin picked up a small mallet and began to pound on the clay mouth he had made. I put my hand to my jaw and made moaning sounds and complained that my teeth were really getting hurt. Martin made no sound but smiled broadly and increased the fervour of his attacks on the clay mouth. Aggressive play with clay mouths continued during the four succeeding sessions. In the fifth session, rather than destroying the clay mouth. Martin fed it a pretend piece of candy. After this he showed no further interest in playing with the clay mouth. In the second session of mouth play he began to speak to the worker, at first behind her back. There were three months of weekly sessions with Martin before school closed. In the late spring Martin began talking with his teacher (p. 70).

Discussion

Parker *et al.* (1960) not only described how the medium of clay was used but they also discussed a number of non-threatening verbal responses which can be used with electively mute children. Specifically, this involved the therapist's describing the patient's nonverbal behavior during assessment and treatment. They outlined a structured sculpturing activity for elective mutism. This involved the therapist's participating in the art process by sculpturing a three-dimensional object which was connected to the elective mutism. This was sufficiently nonthreatening and inviting for the client to participate in the sculpturing activity. Parker *et al.* (1960) also showed how the therapist nonverbally elaborated on the sculpture – i.e., the therapist with his hand on his mouth verbalized his own anxiety about dental appointments. This permitted the patient to express his problem and identify with the therapist.

In the Parker *et al.* (1960) research, the acknowledgement of nonverbal responses occured early in therapy when the patient's communications were limited to nonverbal responses, during intermediate phases when the patient engaged in reluctant speech (e.g., responding when asked a question) and during the phase characterized by spontaneous speech. The study also discusses nonverbal responses which can be used by the therapist (including turning his/her back to the patient) to make it easier for the electively mute person to talk. Specific guidelines including contraindications, however, for using this technique are not provided.

Pustrom and Speers

Study I: Finger-Painting, Story-Telling and Drawing

Pustrom and Speers (1964) described how art therapy was used with an eight-year-old electively mute boy. The child was referred for therapy because he refused to talk to anyone with the exception of a few adults and other children. Although his parents feared that he would not be promoted in school, they assumed that he would outgrow the problem. Their fears were temporarily allayed when he was promoted from the first grade and when it was reported that:

Johnny's second grade teacher was extraordinarily encouraging and coaxed Johnny to read. He condescended to read to her, in a whisper, only if his mother was also present. The teacher reported that he had given up ice cream at school rather than name the flavour he desired (p. 290).

The authors' reported that the client finger-painted freely and typed stories about his paintings. The use of art and story-telling was helpful because it enabled the therapist to interpret the patient's angry feelings toward his mother, and his wishes to control her through his incessant chatter at home.

Study II: Finger-Painting, Story-Telling and Drawing

The second eight-year old boy in the Pustrom and Speers (1964) investigation was also involved in finger-painting, typing stories, and drawing. According to the authors, these techniques enabled the therapist to interpret the child's hostile feelings. On two occasions, within a time span of three years, he was withdrawn from school by the mother. The first occasion was a church nursery school in which he "kicked, screamed, and called for his mother" [and] "when she did not appear, he became quiet and sullen, and withdrew from the other children" (p. 288). Because of this behavior, the mother finally withdrew him from the nursery school.

At age five he entered kindergarten and repeated the same behavior he had exhibited in the nursery school. He was withdrawn from school after six months because of tonsillitis. He entered grade one at age six but the problems of separation were more difficult than in either the nursery school or kindergarten. The patient's mother dealt with his school refusal by entering the classroom but leaving her son when his back was turned. Each time he discovered that his mother had left the room, he became rigid, hung his head, and refused to look at people in the room. At the time of referral, he would talk only to his family and to a few children on the playground. The patient's written work was satisfactory and so he was promoted. The client's mother repeatedly cautioned the child not to talk to his paternal grandmother because he might divulge family secrets to her which she, in turn, might tell her own therapist.

The therapist's permissiveness enabled the child to express his hostility about the mother through a dream report. In the first dream, the mother was dead and in a second dream the boy's female cat had been decapitated. There is no explanation, however, of the role played by these two dreams in the child's acquisition of speech refusal or the child's treatment. Initially, the mother accompanied the patient to the classroom. There followed a progressively increasing distance at which his mother would leave him before he entered the school. Similarly, the onset time of his silence increased prior to therapy sessions. Initially, he became silent when he and his mother entered the automobile to go to the clinic. The onset of the silence gradually occurred at a progressively shorter distance from the therapist's office. Finally, the patient began talking in the waiting room and only became silent when he entered the playroom. At the conclusion of therapy, he was speaking to everyone but his therapist.

Study III: Play Therapy and Finger-Painting

An eight-year old girl (Pustrom and Speers, 1964) was referred for treatment by her parents because of non-talking and social withdrawal. The father's approach to the problem was primarily passive but he did attempt to bribe the child into talking to him. In spite of this, she talked very little to her father. The mother, on the other hand, insisted she do the talking for her children to reduce the likelihood of their saying something wrong. The client's mother disliked being asked questions and often took over conversations to avoid being asked questions. When the patient was four years old they lived in a small town in Central America and the children of the village treated the patient and her brothers as "unwelcome outsiders." At that time the mother returned to the States, thus separating herself and the children from the father. During the next two years the family moved several times. The child began kindergarten at age five and regular school the following year. She spoke to neither the other children nor the teachers.

Therapy consisted of two components. First, doll play was used to enact a dream:

In doll play, with the therapist verbalizing the various roles and pointing out the unhappiness [death wishes and guilt] the silent child suffered, resulting in considerable change in Gwen's overall behavior. Gwen began talking with her teacher and with other female adults. She showed some desire to separate from her overprotective mother by joining a Brownie group, and specifically requesting that her mother not participate in this activity. To her therapist, she began showing considerable aggression, but was unable to talk to him (Pustrom and Speers, 1964, p. 295).

The second component of the therapy was finger-painting. According to the authors:

Her finger-painting activity invariably produced a girl named "Susan" whom Gwen desired to emulate. Susan's mouth was always painted as "open." The therapist interpreted Gwen's desire to be like Susan and suggested she could attain this wish (Pustrom and Speers, 1964, p. 295).

Discussion

In the Pustrom and Speers investigation, samples or descriptions of the children's finger-paintings and typewritten stories were not provided. Although the finger-paintings and story-writing were mentioned in the discussion of treatment, they were not the major variables in treatment. Both art and story-telling offer an abundance of therapeutic opportunities. The children could have been encouraged to change their stories to reveal effective coping skills for a more favorable outcome. This might have occurred during unstructured finger-drawing and story-telling with direct therapist participation in both of these activities. I suggest that the participation of the therapist in these two activities might be called mutual finger painting and mutual story-telling. Mutual story-telling, however, is not new; it refers to a well-known technique developed by Gardner (1971). Concerning the second eight-year-old boy, nothing is mentioned about the process of the art activities such as time invested, sequence in which the images were drawn, or the developmental characteristics of the child's drawings. These activities gave the therapist an excellent opportunity to assess the patient's nonverbal communication but since the major variable was speaking, minimal information is reported about the development of nonverbal behavior.

The Pustrom and Speers (1964) clinical investigation is significant because none of these children talked to the therapist, yet they talked to other persons at the conclusion of treatment. The authors interpreted the children's failure to speak to the therapist as a last-ditch stand against giving up manipulative control of others. One can speculate that in future stressful situations the children might revert to their stubborn silence.

Mora, Spencer, DeVault and Schopler

Mora *et al.* (1962) studied electively mute twins who had not spoken for seven years. They were enrolled in the second semester of grade six at the time of their referral. The authors reported that the first time that the twins' mutism was observed was at the age of three when their paternal grandmother was looking after them for ten days. The mother attributed their silence to shyness and she said that she "often did not feel like talking herself if an unpleasant subject was brought up, but didn't have the courage of the girls not to talk" (p. 42).

Separate class placement for each twin was not successful in eliciting speech. The twins employed a form of sign language to communicate with each other when other children were present and if a stranger addressed them, they looked at each other as if they had a pact to remain silent. When asked *why they elected to be silent*, Joyce wrote:

When I was small, I didn't want to talk for some reason I don't know. Now I am older, I still don't know. I am afraid of what other people will say if I start now. Without first talking to her sister, Ruth wrote: "My reason is the same reason why my sister didn't talk. She didn't talk so I didn't talk. I don't know the reason (p. 42).

In this investigation, two therapists were assigned to each patient to promote a healthy separation from the mother and also to assist in developing a separate identity for the twins. Each twin remained mute while being assessed with the WISC but cooperated by writing their responses. Intelligence was estimated to be 98 and 94 for Ruth and Joyce respectively. Although neither twin spoke, each drew pictures when asked. Ruth drew a girl resembling herself, seen from the front but turning her head away, her hands behind her back and with considerable erasing around the mouth. The authors reported that Ruth's drawings indicated that she was aware of her problem of speech refusal. They also said that Ruth was more involved with her own independence and with adolescent problems than was her twin.

Joyce painted a house, sketching a fence around it heavily with black paint, the whole scene being rather lifeless. According to the authors, Joyce's picture suggested that she seemed concerned with hiding herself and shutting out people and the world. They also claimed that Joyce appeared immature and was more dependent than her twin on home and family.

Phase One: Therapeutic Relationship

The first phase of treatment might be called "relationship building." The authors reported that certain unspecified games were played – presumably requiring nonverbal rather than verbal responses. Both clients remained mute during the games. Toward the end of this phase, the authors reported that each of the twins was becoming more relaxed as suggested by smiling and occasionally laughing.

Phase Two: Story-Telling and Drawing

The second phase of treatment also focused on nonverbal communication. The authors attempted to obtain information about the specific symptom of elective mutism as well as about other problems which the adolescents might be experiencing. They used a customized Kent-Rosanoff Word Association List with words interpolated which had special relevance to speech refusal. In addition, several TAT cards were used and the girls were asked to write stories about these. The particular TAT cards which were used to elicit stories were not indicated. The patient's written responses revealed that Joyce was self-conscious about being "made fun of" and she also seemed more prone to denial, to running away from difficulties and hiding her feelings than Ruth.

Patient drawings were again introduced during this phase. Each girl independently drew a house. Ruth drew a house in pencil, a simple house but refused to elaborate about it. Joyce's house, on the other hand, was also a front view but was comprised of two units, almost as a "twin house." Joyce elaborated as follows:

My house. I don't like it because the colors are horrible, and it is old and the trimmings need painting. Otherwise, it is a nice house (p. 44).

The authors claimed that the patients' house drawings supported their hypothesis that Ruth seemed more concerned with individuality and Joyce with twinship.

Phase Three: Expressions in Writing, Clay and Drawings

During this phase, Mora *et al.* (1962) reported that the patients were questioned specifically about their symptoms, coming for treatment and about being a twin. Joyce expressed concern about coming for treatment. Both shared a dislike of each other and of being pressured or pushed. Once written communication was begun, the therapists felt less uneasy about the lack of speech. The therapist suggested that Ruth appeared angry and she agreed. Ruth was told that she was afraid of expressing anger. Later, while Ruth was *manipulating some clay*, the therapist told Ruth that she felt like throwing something at him. This statement did not elicit a comment from the client. At the therapist's suggestion, Ruth made a drawing. It depicted:

. . . a slender, teenaged girl, blonde, with a long red dress and again, her hands behind her back. This girl was wearing lipstick and had long hair (p. 45).

According to her two therapists, the drawing seemed to emphasize the oral aspects of sexuality while denying the genital ones. Joyce seemed to be afraid to be independent and was ambivalent and jealous about Ruth – especially threatening was Ruth's boyfriend who might contribute to separating her from her twin. Hostility and frustration were exhibited by Joyce's shooting a toy gun during an entire session.

During this same period, therapy with the mother focused on her role in the elective mutism of the twins. According to Mora *et al.* (1962), she seemed to inadvertently foster a dependency relationship between the twins in two ways: first, by threats of "separating them for good" if they misbehaved toward each other and, second, by exerting pressure to keep the twins together by encouraging each to include the other in her activities. Joyce, at this stage was beginning to express fantasies about teen-age activities, which included showing the therapist her pictures of rock-and-roll singers.

When the fear of separation between the twins had subsided, the newly achieved sense of individual identity was tested by a separate camp placement for each for two weeks during the summer. The twins had never been separated before. In her writing, Ruth expressed a firm determination not to go to camp, because she believed that camp was for "crazy people" and she also feared that the activities in camp might be geared for younger children. Nonetheless, Ruth actively participated in camp; she made friends and talked freely, although she did not speak to the director. Joyce, on the other hand, talked with only a few girls but was active in the scheduled activities. Both girls were well liked.

Phase Four: Directive to Talk

The school principal had been informed of the progress to date, and he communicated to the mother and children that he expected them to talk or leave school. The reaction of the girls was to talk as little as possible in school but gradually they began to orally participate in class. Their school participation increased and by the end of the year, Ruth was on the honor roll and Joyce passed all her courses. The disappearance of the symptoms reduced the urgency for treatment and, by agreement, treatments were more widely spaced.

Discussion

In the Mora *et al.* (1962) investigation, the client differentiated experiences coming before and after treatment and she indicated that she:

recognized her previous neurotic behavior as "silly." She said she felt "funny," not being able to talk to some people she had known for a long time, while she felt quite comfortable in talking to people who didn't know her. She added that if she talked freely to people who had known her, "they would tell me how silly and everything I was [before treatment]" (p. 47).

The drawings seemed to have played a minimal role in assessment and it is not clear if the drawings had a "therapeutic-healing" function.

CHAPTER 22

EXPRESSIVE THERAPY INTERVENTIONS
PART 2

PLAY THERAPY

Lesser-Katz (1988) does not abandon words completely during play therapy even though the electively mute person does not reciprocate by talking. The therapist's spoken words are directed at interpreting the child's feelings. The children whom she studied were found to demonstrate greater mastery over their feelings and a greater sense of security once they learned to express feelings with words. Lesser-Katz (1988) claimed that through the use of words, one does not have to resort to defenses like denial and other avoidance strategies to master the expression of affect.

USE OF LETTERS

Krolian (1988) reported that when the seven-year-old female she treated refused to enter her office, she wrote and delivered a letter to the child. The author reported that this process eased the child's anxieties, reduced the child's fear of intrusiveness, and created an accepting environment for the child.

USE OF THE TELEPHONE IN TREATING ELECTIVE MUTISM

Krolian (1988) indicated that her female client also showed an interest in dialing random numbers on the telephone. She instructed the child to dial the number for a recorded message for the weather and time. In the second phase, the therapist went to an adjoining office and suggested that the client telephone her. To this request, the child nodded agreement and dialed the therapist. The child unintelligibly whispered answers to the therapist's questions, blew a whistle into the receiver and slammed the receiver on the desk. The therapist acknowledged these behaviors by commenting that she could hear the different sounds.

PLAY THERAPY CONTENT AND PROCESS

Lesser-Katz (1988) treated elective mutism in the setting where the problem occurred – the school. The researcher indicated that she first played briefly with the other children and then involved some of them as peer counsellors. Lesser-Katz described the process and outcome of each step of her intervention. During *Phases 1 and 2*, the client did not communicate either verbally or nonverbally. The therapist tried asking questions which could have been answered by nodding, but the client did not reply. The mother indicated that the client responded positively to the therapist but was unable to provide examples of specific behaviors to support her statement. In *Phase 3*, the therapist engaged the client in rolling one car back and forth. After the client had predictably demonstrated compliance with the therapist's request, she introduced a second car. At the conclusion of the session, the therapist asked the client if he would like something to eat. The client nodded affirmatively. This was his first gesture which conformed to nonverbal communication. In *Phase 4*, the therapist instructed the child to say "Go" whenever he wanted her to roll the car. The client complied but in a barely audible voice. Subsequently, the therapist asked the client to say "Go fast" when he wanted her to quickly roll the car. Again the client complied but spoke in a whisper.

In the *5th Phase* the client responded *gesturally with "Yes" and "No."* During the *6th Phase,* the child complied by playing with two peer helpers. The client repeated in the presence of others what the therapist had asked him to say which was a brief request to his teacher to leave the classroom with the therapist. The child said that he enjoyed playing, but became mute again when his mother entered the room. During *Phases 7 and 8* the client joined the therapist in a rocking chair shaped like a boat. Smooth and rhythmic motions were facilitated by the boat-rocking play. The structure of the toy itself lessened what the therapist described as the "wooden" movements of the client. The activity was later accompanied by the client repeating phrases sung by the therapist. In the *final phase* the client played hide-and-seek with the therapist. According to the therapist the game was accompanied by noticeable facial animation. At this time, the client stopped talking to the therapist for about a month. The teacher reported, however, that he was leading his class during some activities and would answer some questions with a nodding gesture. Disinhibition of saying certain words followed. Other children were involved in taking turns saying "bad words." According to Lesser-Katz (1988), the client would say these types of words (e.g., pee-pee) in a clear and explicit manner.

DANCE AND MOVEMENT THERAPY

Communication involves behavior expressed through sounds, intonations, postures and gestures. Schmerling and Kerins (1987) emphasized that employing a speech-language therapist in the treatment of elective mutism was a unique approach because speech therapists generally do not work with silence users. Speech therapy was used to establish pre-verbal and verbal communication skills. Dance therapy was used as part of the treatment to help the child to develop meaningful and appropriate expressive behaviors and to foster the child's development of interpersonal relationships.

According to the authors, the combined approach allows the symptoms and the conflicts associated with elective mutism to be addressed. Furthermore, the clients are confronted about their speech refusal and therefore they become fully aware that speech is expected. In this study, the focus was on a series of manageable speech tasks in order to rebuild verbal behavior. The intervention establishes a relationship on a non-verbal level through a variety of dance and movement interactions. An advantage of these activities is that they do not challenge the child's desire to remain silent.

MUSIC THERAPY

Krolian (1988) used music improvision as part of her intervention. The therapist and client made a tape recording of their playing recorders together. This activity involved the making of music, listening to music and presumably responding to each other's music with music. Krolian's approach involved the same modality as the behavior problem. Indeed, speaking involves the auditory modality as does making and listening to music. This approach was probably less threatening for the child than speaking, yet led to her producing sounds in the presence of the therapist.

PET-FACILITATED THERAPY

In contrast to the majority of the published reports of therapeutic interventions, there is only one case study (Roberts, 1984) dealing with pet-facilitated therapy. Roberts (1984) discusses how pets were used in the assessment and treatment of the electively mute behavior of a 14-year-old patient. Her observations and reflections about a pet dog included a number of parallels between the behavior of the pet and the adolescent patient's behavior.

Some of the reframing that we did around Sara's symptom revolved around a wonderful story that emerged in the fourth session when I asked them how their dog Rebel got his name. Ever since I had met Rebel at their house, his name had been troubling me as it just did not fit into the language of this very protective family which did not disagree, take stands on one's own, or "rebel" in any way. It turned out that Rebel had been taken in by Mr. Y after a coworker had to get rid of him. Upon bringing Rebel home, they changed his name to Bubbles (it fits!) but Rebel was stubborn and would not come to anything but his first name so they went back to it. As Sara was very attached to dogs (she had her own dog that she named Rocky but the family called Baby), I used this story to connote some of Sara's behavior as stubborn in the same way Rebel had been stubborn (Roberts, 1984, p. 44).

Based on the adolescent's interest in animals, the parents were asked to buy a pet parakeet. Roberts and her colleagues had the patient privately make tape recordings for the bird, saying the same word a number of times for the bird to repeat. The patient's and the bird's vocabulary were monitored and as the vocabulary of each increased, the clinicians played the recorded messages for family members and then to the people at the treatment centre. At the conclusion of treatment, Roberts (1984) reported that the child was talking to family members on the telephone. Furthermore, she was observed talking to family members in face-to-face conversations.

PET-FACILITATED THERAPY

Note[22.1]

Introduction

"Pet-facilitated therapy refers to integrating animals into client directed activities" (Brickel, 1986, p. 309). The use of pets in the therapeutic process does not depend on the theoretical orientation of the clinician. It depends instead on the ingenuity of the therapist.

According to Levinson (cited in Ross, 1983) there are a number of advantages of using pets as adjuncts to therapy.

The importance of the pet to man is psychological, not practical. The relationship between humans and animals can oft-times be more salutary than between two humans. A pet can satisfy a human's needs for loyalty, trust and respect. A relationship with an animal can be less threatening than a relationship with a human. Animals are alive and, as such, provide greater therapeutic opportunities than play toys. The arena in which one would work with child and animal is much broader than a therapist's office. Animals can speed up the therapeutic process. Animals can be around 24 hours a day if they are needed. (p. 32)

Brickel (1981) argues that pets are suitable for psychotherapeutic roles because they are "fascinating to watch" and are capable of "serving as companions." The ability of pets to give "affection and comfort" is well understood by pet owners. Their dependency instills a "sense of responsibility" and "self esteem." Furthermore, they serve as a useful "catalyst for social interaction" (p. 120). Of particular significance for elective mutism is the study by Corson and Corson (1990). They claim that one individual who had been mute for 26 years spoke his first words when PFT became a part of his treatment. Pets also serve an important role in fostering the physical health of pet owners. For example, weight loss through exercising a pet has been associated with involvement in a PFT program (Corson and Corson, 1990).

In implementing PFT one needs to consider three major factors. These are: (1) the selection of the therapist, (2) the selection of the client who will benefit from the presence of a pet, and (3) the selection of the pet.

Selection of the Therapist

The therapist should be one who enjoys animals – although he or she does not have to own a pet to be considered appropriate for the role. The therapist will be responsible for the well-being of the patient and the pet. The therapist should also demonstrate patience and flexibility in dealing with animals because animals, like people, can be uncooperative. The person selected to implement PFT should also show a measure of creativity because he or she will have to integrate PFT into the theoretical rationale of the intervention. If the therapist is a behaviourist the person will probably want to integrate the PFT into a reinforcement framework, if the therapist takes a psychodynamic approach, the person may wish to integrate the PFT into the part of the therapeutic rationale which addresses symbolic content and if the therapist favours a reality therapy orientation he may wish to include PFT into a responsibility focus. (Brickel, 1986)

Selection of Clients

Another important issue is selecting the clients who will benefit from PFT. I cannot give you any definitive statement about this but the standard guidelines at present indicate that PFT is contraindicated for clients who are allergic to animals or fearful of animals. If the clients' fear is limited to specific animals (e.g., dogs), then one might still be able to use PFT if one does not use a dog as a "co-therapist." PFT is also contraindicated for clients who have a history of "acting out" and who have a history of being cruel to animals. As part of an initial assessment, the client might be given a stuffed toy animal (Brickel, 1981). The toy animal may be therapeutic (Francis and Baly, 1984) but the intent here is to monitor the client's reaction to the stuffed toy animal.

Selection of the Pet

The task of selecting the pet is as important as selecting the therapist who will use the animal in PFT, the real or anticipated reactions of the staff, and the selection of the clients who are likely to benefit from PFT. One factor which needs to be considered is the age of the animal. Mature animals are preferable to young animals because:

- older animals are housebroken.
- the use of mature animals may reduce the pet's bonding to one person.
- the size of the animal is an important factor especially if one intends to introduce PFT into a crowded facility; if a mature animal is used the size is already established and therefore it is easier to make a judgement about the suitability of the animal.

There are also special considerations which relate to the well-being of the animal which is selected to serve as an adjunct to therapy. Two of these special considerations include:

- providing the pet with access to a protected setting in which to relax; children can make continuous demands on pets and therefore it is in the pet's interest that it be given a quiet place to which the children do not have access.
- monitoring of overfeeding which may put the pet at risk for illness.

Placing a Pet in the Home

According to Brickel in his reviews of PFT, pets can serve as companions in the homes of clients. He cautions, however, that this option should be thoroughly considered because if the client is retired or on a meagre disability allowance he or she may not be able to afford the pet unless a source of funding is found for the support of the pet. The additional economic burden may even outweigh the physiological and psychological advantages of having the person-pet companionship. Before placing a pet in the person's home one would also want to determine if the person is physically able to care for the animal and if the person is available to care for the pet. (A person whose work required him or her to be away may find caring for the pet burdensome even though there were positive features in having a companion in the home). These obstacles are not unsurmountable but they need to be recognized and addressed. The issue of care in a residential setting, however, presents a different set of circumstances. For example, if an elderly person in a nursing home is unable to care for the animal other patients or staff could be asked to volunteer to do this.

Potential Negative Staff Reactions

There are several potential negative reactions of pet-facilitated therapy. Negative responses from staff may relate to five major areas. These are:

- the fear of spreading disease.
- a decrement in the quality and delivery of medical services.
- legal concerns (especially if a patient were injured by a pet).
- allergic reactions of staff and patients to the presence of the pets.
- the "clashing" of PFT with interventions based on "traditional models." One approach which may reduce the negative reactions is to use staff volunteers to monitor the effects of the PFT and if need be to care for the pets. If the staff objects to multiple pets it is recommended to carefully select one animal and to use it as the "mascot" for the setting (Brickel, 1981).

Potential Positive Staff Reactions

According to Brickel (1981) one may anticipate positive reactions because:

- the staff may be encouraged by the patient's reactions to the animals (e.g., smiling and other nonverbal behaviours) and other observable changes in the client's behaviour (e.g., increase in intelligible speech).
- the staff may report that the environment is less cold and sterile. The presence of pets brings a "naturalness" to the setting.
- the staff may enjoy having pets or a mascot in the setting. The animals may provide needed occasional "positive diversions" from the professional duties of the staff – without interfering with the quality and delivery of medical services.

STORY-TELLING AND PET-FACILITATED THERAPY

Southworth (1987) outlines her encounter with an electively mute child in the *Cambridge Journal of Education*. Despite the therapist's determination to make the student talk the teacher was unable to do so. Apparently the child did talk the previous year but because the teacher moved to another school, the therapist was unable to determine what the teacher did to elicit speech. Although the child was seen by a number of professionals, the nature and progress of specific treatments were not detailed. No one had observed the child talking or responding to teacher questions in his three years at school although he had been observed making a few animal noises to children.

Phase 1 of treatment involved the therapist's writing notes to the parents and vice versa. Recordings were made of the child's reading to his parents at home and the audiotape was periodically returned to the school so that the teacher would have an opportunity of hearing the child talk. The teacher continued to use the tape recorder and, in addition, asked if the child would let her play the tape to the class so that his peers would hear what his voice was like. The child gave his consent to play the tape to his agemates. Prior to playing the tape, the teacher prepared the class by prompting them to applaud the tape when it was played in class.

The contact with the parents via the "communication book" and audiotape permitted therapy to be monitored. The "disclosure" of his voice to his agemates was accompanied by a number of brief talking episodes in the vicinity of his home. For example, the child was observed speaking for the first time to his brother's friends. Furthermore, the client also observed his mother talking to his teacher in a setting (i.e., the school) in which he exhibited speech refusal. The "communication book" revealed that the child had a pet dog. The teacher asked the client on the tape if he would tell the class on the tape about his pet. This was his first episode of spontaneous speech and he permitted the tape to be played to his classmates.

Phase 2: Nonverbally Responding to Questions. The tape was played to the class and he replied to questions from the class about his puppy by nodding his head for an affirmative response and turning his head from side-to-side for a negative response.

Phase 3: Mouthing "YES" and "NO." He complied with the teacher's request to mouth "yes" and "no" to answer questions.

Phase 4: Animal Sounds on Request. In this phase, the teacher asked the child to make the barking sound of his puppy. He again complied.

Phase 5: Client-Initiated Speech. This phase involved client-initiated speech at school. After hearing a talk on safety, the child's best friend reported to the teacher that he had observed the client say, "I wouldn't want to be electrocuted."

Phase 6: Whispering. This phase was also client-initiated; whispering later generalized to other teachers.

Discussion

The Southworth (1987) article is one of the very few in the elective mutism literature to address the issue of why electively mute individuals begin to speak. The teacher-therapist identified a number of potential, nonspecific treatment factors which may have been operating in isolation or in combination.

- Mother-teacher contact and the more relaxed approach to his problem which resulted. I would also add that since he spontaneously spoke to his mother at home that the mother was a natural cue to speak. The fact that his mother was present in the classroom may have helped to transform the classroom into a setting where it was safe to speak.
- By permitting the tape recorder to be played in the classroom while alone with the teacher, he undoubtedly observed that it was also safe to play the tape recorder in classroom setting in the presence of the other children.
- The handwritten notes involved a more personal approach than typewritten letters.
- The child's puppy provided a topic and an incentive for the child to communicate to the class (p. 158).

Client self-reports and interviews with the parents and friends would have readily provided a data base for these hypotheses. Such interviews would have also given the client and his family an opportunity to reflect on the therapeutic process and to generate their own hypotheses. In other words, it may have been helpful in identifying treatment variables if both the young client and family members were asked to explain their perceptions of his initiating speech with non-family members at home and to the teachers and children at school.

This study is extremely systematic and clear in its description of the treatment. In addition, potential independent variables are clearly delineated. Potential reinforcers, however, are not identified, although it is easy to conjecture that client self-reinforcement may have been involved. I am especially thinking of the young client hearing his own voice and telling something to the other children that he wanted to tell. The positive response of the other children when the teacher first played the tape of the child reading to his parents at home and the applause of the class after the teacher played the tape seems to be an identifiable positive event which may have been positively reinforcing for the child. And we must not forget about the teacher's praise which undoubtedly was positively reinforcing. Note especially the mention of "smiles" and "drawing him close" which were referred to in the article. The teacher set up a hierarchy of speaking situations and the child complied by exposing himself to successively more-and-more anxiety arousing situations. The graduated series of "reality-testing" tasks perhaps contributed to extinguishing the speaking fears.

PERSON-FOCUSED DRAMA THERAPY

In the Ciottone and Madonna (1984) investigation, there was a naturalness about the sequence of events which occurred during therapy. The

11-year-old client established his own hierarchy of communication events and progressed through the hierarchy at his own rate. The client-initiated hierarchy progressed from academic-focused communication (doing and correcting mathematics problems) to gradually more communication-focused responses beginning with writing teachers' names on the chalkboard, to writing narratives on the chalkboard and ending with typing statements about the activities of the group. In the final phase of the client-initiated exposure to communication contexts, the client began to write questions on the board which had been addressed to him by the therapist and peers. At about the same time, he progressed to writing questions and messages to the therapist and peers. Up to this point, however, the client rarely verbalized. *The abrupt transition to verbal communication was marked by the client's seizing the microphone from the therapist and by the client's improvising the content of an interview scenario.*

Discussion

The child in the Ciottone and Madonna (1984) investigation elected to communicate by writing on the chalkboard and by typing messages. In the final phase of treatment, the client seized control of an interview scenario and seems to have individualized his communication during the improvisation. The authors do not refer to this as drama therapy nor do they report the "before" and "after" nonverbal behaviors which were associated with the silence user role and the active speaking role of the client. Nor do the authors attempt to account for the child's speaking during the interview scene. It is not necessary, however, to refer to the theory, research and practice of drama therapy in order to offer a plausible explanation for the client's speaking. A parallel exists in the literature on stuttering dating to the publication of Van Riper (1971). It has been observed that individuals do not stutter when singing or when using an accent or dialect which is not their own. It seems likely, therefore, that the "drama therapy" component permitted the client to assume an "acting role," – a make-believe role, which was in contrast to the silence user role. The effect of the "drama therapy" could also be given a behavioral interpretation. Self-modeling in which people with problems serve as their own positive model occurred naturally during the brief drama therapy phase of the treatment. This may account for the maintenance of his verbal behavior but it does not account for his initially emitting verbal behavior because speaking occurred at the same time as the positive self-modeling experience. Ordinarily for self-modeling to operate, the model of desired behavior must precede the patient's emitting the desired behavior.

Unfortunately, a description of the verbal and nonverbal communication of the client was not included in the clinical report. The main focus was on molar description, that is on the intent or "what" of the behavior.

Molecular description, however, would have answered "how" questions about the client's communication because molecular description include photographic-like details.

Self-modeling therapy is based on Bandura's (1986) social cognitive theory. According to self-modeling theory, behavior change is produced by self-efficacy. Kehle *et al.* (1990) sum up the relevance of self-modeling as an intervention for elective mutism. They claim that:

Self-modeling alters efficacy beliefs, which in turn change performance. If this line of reasoning is valid, then elective mute children, through viewing edited videotapes depicting themselves talking in a classroom situation, learn to believe that they can successfully communicate with their peers and teachers, and subsequently behave in accordance with that belief, and are reinforced for doing so (p. 120).

One might speculate that unplanned-for self-modeling occurred in the Ciottone and Madonna (1984) study. If a video-recording had been made of the interview scenario in the Ciottone and Madonna study, and if the client observed himself talking in the setting in which he elected to be silent, the approach would have been similar to the Kehle *et al.* procedure.

If the client later verbalized the details of his verbal and nonverbal behavior during the scenario, this would indicate that the client recognized that he spoke during the interview scenario. If the client were able to retain a tactile-kinesthetic memory of seizing the microphone and holding it while speaking, an auditory memory for the content of his verbal behavior and a visual memory of speaking in the setting where he elected to be silent, one could argue for naturally occurring positive self-modeling. Presumably, the consequences for speaking were positive and this means that the therapeutic effect might be explained by a combination of self-modeling and positive reinforcement. The client's imitation of the interview scenario may also have modified the statements that the client said to himself about himself (e.g., "I do talk here" instead of self-defeating statements such as "I do not talk here").

Up to this point, I have discussed a multi-sensory learning experience which parallels the multi-sensory remedial procedures such as the V-isual, A-uditory, K-inesthetic and T-actile procedure of Fernald (1943). Fernald's work is discussed in the majority of the survey texts in learning disabilities. It is tempting to hypothesize that the multi-sensory experience of the presumed positive-self-modeling contributed to the client's talking in the setting in which he elected to be silent. To my knowledge, the role of the sensory modalities in positive self-modeling has not been investigated. This would not be a difficult task. Manipulating the videotape feedback would enable the impact of the audio component, the visual component and the combined visual and the auditory component to be assessed.

CEREMONY IN TREATING ELECTIVE MUTISM

Ceremony and ritual was employed at the conclusion of the treatment of a 14-year-old adolescent to celebrate the success of treatment and to symbolize the burying of the mutistic response in an investigation by Roberts (1984). The clinical team and the adolescent client buried a metal box covered with birds because of their role in getting the adolescent to talk. The box was buried on the grounds of the hospital in case the client needed it again if she stopped talking. According to Roberts (1984), this is what happened during the ceremony:

Sara was asked to pick a spot on the grounds to bury the box, and with her father she sighted several landmarks so as to have a place where it could be found again. Gathering in a circle, we all took turns shovelling out a hole. I then placed the box in the hole and asked each person to comment on what they wanted to say to each other about the future as they put a shovelful of dirt over the past. The comments centered around never having to dig the box up, pleasure in Sara's coming home and thanks to the treatment center (p. 51).

STORY-TELLING AND BIBLIOTHERAPY

Story-telling is recommended by Friedman and Karagan (1973) as an approach which can be used by parents and teachers. A more systematic approach, however, is bibliotherapy in which the story-teller carefully selects age-appropriate stories which are related to elective mutism. The book *Helping Children Cope* by Fassler (1978) reviews children's literature and suggests how books and stories can be used to reduce fears and initiate communication. Stories to help children counteract the fear of abandonment and the separation-type stories that relate to early school experiences are worth considering for electively mute children especially if these issues are suspected to be contributing to elective mutism. Several of the books which Fassler recommended are listed below:

Reassuring Stories to Help Counteract Fears of Abandonment

- Brown, M.W. (1942). *The Runaway Bunny*. New York: Harper & Row.
- Krauss, R. (1951). *The Bundle Book*. New York: Harper & Row.
- Schlein, M. (1963). *The Way Mothers Are*. Chicago: Albert Whitman.

Separation Stories Related to Early School Experiences

- Blue, R. (1971). *I Am Here: Yo Estoy Aqui*. New York: Franklin Watts.
- Breinburg, P. (1973) *Shawn Goes to School*. New York: Thomas Y. Crowell.

- Cohen, M. (1967). *Will I Have a Friend?* New York: Collier.
- Katzoff, B. (1964). *Cathy's First School.* New York: Alfred A. Knopf.
- Mannheim, G. (1968). *The Two Friends.* New York: Alfred A. Knopf.
- Steiner, C. (1965). *I'd Rather Stay With You.* New York: Seabury Press.
- Thayer, J. (1963). *A Drink For Little Red Diker.* New York: William Morrow.
- Yashima, T. (1958). *Umbrella.* New York: Viking Press.

Separation from Parents for Reasons Not Related to School Activities

- Brown, M.B. (1960). *First Night Away from Home.* New York: Franklin Watts.
- Chalmers, M. (1967). *Be Good Harry.* New York: Harper & Row.
- Waber, B. (1972). *Ira Sleeps Over.* Boston: Houghton Mifflin.

Accidental Separation from a Parent or Parent-Figure

- McCloskey, R. (1948). *Blueberries for Sal.* New York: Viking Press.
- Reyher, B. (1945). *My Mother Is the Most Beautiful Woman in the World.* New York: Lothrop, Lee & Sheppard.
- Vogel, Ilse-Margaret (1965). *Hello Henry.* New York: Parents' Magazine Press.

Separation from a Well-Liked and Trusted Individual

- Cohen, M. (1972). *The New Teacher.* New York: Macmillan.
- Minarik, E.H. (1960). *Little Bear's Friend.* New York: Harper & Row
- Simon, N. (1965). *Benjy's Bird.* Chicago: Albert Whitman.
- Steig, W. (1971). *Amos and Boris.* New York: Farrar, Straus & Giroux.

Discussion

The above sources deal primarily with characteristics which may be linked to elective mutism. The therapist, however, may elect to prepare a story which directly aligns with the particular characteristics of his or her client's use of silence. The child in the custom-prepared story should depict a coping rather than a fearless model. Specific guidelines for story construction include coping skills for speaking fears, advantages of speaking in the target setting and a positive outcome showing a transition from silence to spontaneous speech.

REFERENCES

Achenbach, T.M. (1978). *Research in Developmental Psychology: Concepts, Strategies, Methods.* New York: Free Press.

Adams, M. and Glasser, J. (1954). Emotional involvements in some forms of mutism. *Journal of Speech and Hearing Disorders* 19, 56–60.

Albert-Stewart, P.L. (1986). Positive reinforcement in short-term treatment of an electively mute child: A case study. *Psychological Reports* 58, 571–576.

Alberto, P.A. and Troutman, A.C. (1986). *Applied Behavior Analysis for Teachers.* Columbus, OH: Merrill.

Alexander, C. (1979). *The Timeless Way of Building.* New York: Oxford University Press.

Ambrosino, S.V. and Alessi, M. (1979). Elective mutism: Fixation and the double bind. *The American Journal of Psychoanalysis* 39, 251–256.

American Psychiatric Association. (1987). *Diagnostic and Statistical Manual of Mental Disorders* (3rd ed., revised). Washington, DC: American Psychiatric Association.

American Psychiatric Association. (1991). *DSM–IV Option's Book.* Washington, DC: American Psychiatric Association.

Appelman, K., Allen, K.E. and Turner, K.D. (1975). The conditioning of language in a non-verbal child conducted in a special education classroom. *Journal of Speech and Hearing Disorders* 40, 3–12.

Atkinson, J.M. and Heritage, J. (eds.) (1984). *Structure of Social Action: Studies in Conversation Analysis.* New York: Cambridge University Press.

Atoynatan T.H. (1986). Elective mutism: Involvement of the mother in the treatment of the child. *Child Psychiatry and Human Development* 17, 15–27.

Axelrod, S. (1983). *Behavior Modification for the Classroom Teacher* (2nd ed.). New York: McGraw-Hill.

Ayllon, T. and Kelly, K. (1974). Reinstating verbal behavior in a functionally mute retardate. *Professional Psychology* 5, 385–393.

Babbitt, R.L. and Parrish, J.M. (1991). Phone phobia, phact or phantasy?: An operant approach to a child's disruptive behavior induced by telephone usage. *Journal of Behavior Therapy and Experimental Psychiatry* 22, 123–129.

Baldwin, J. (1968). *Tell Me How Long the Train's Been Gone.* New York: Dial.

Bandler, R. and Grinder, J. (1975). *The Structure of Magic: A Book about Language and Therapy* (Vol. 1). Palo Alto, CA: Science and Behavior Books.

Bandura, A. (1986). *Social Foundations of Thought and Action: A Social-Cognitive Theory.* Englewood Cliffs, NJ: Prentice-Hall.

Barbara, D.A. (1958). *The Art of Listening.* Springfield, IL: Charles C. Thomas.

Barlow, D.H. and Hayes, S.C. (1979). Alternating treatment design: One strategy for comparing the effects of two treatments in a single subject. *Journal of Applied Behavior Analysis* 12, 199–210.

Barlow, D.H., Hayes, S.C. and Nelson, R.O. (1984). *The Scientist Practitioner.* New York: Pergamon Press.

Barlow, D.H. and Hersen, M. (1984). *Single Case Experimental Design: Strategies for Studying Behavior* (2nd ed.). New York: Pergamon Press.

Barlow, K., Strother, J. and Landreth, G. (1986). Sibling group play therapy: An effective alternative with an elective mute child. *The School Counselor* 34, 44–50.

221

Bauermeister, J.J. and Jemail, J.A. (1975). Modification of "elective mutism" in the classroom setting: A case study. *Behavior Therapy* 6, 246–250.

Bauman, R. (1983). *Let Your Words Be Few: Symbolism of Speaking and Silence among Seventeenth-Century Quakers*. New York: Cambridge University Press.

Bausell, R.B. (1991). *Advanced Research Methodology: An Annotated Guide to Sources*. Metuchen, NJ: Scarecrow Press.

Beattie, G.W. (1978). Floor apportionment and gaze in conversational dyads. *British Journal of Social and Clinical Psychology* 17, 7–15.

Beattie, G.W. (1979). Contextual constraints on the floor-apportionment function of speaker-gaze in dyadic conversations. *British Journal of Social and Clinical Psychology* 18, 391–392.

Beattie, G.W. (1981a). The regulation of speaker turns in face-to-face conversations: Some implications for conversation in sound-only communication channels. *Semiotica* 34, 55–70.

Beattie, G.W. (1981b). A further investigation of the cognitive interference hypothesis of gaze patterns during conversation. *British Journal of Social Psychology* 20, 243–348.

Beck, J.R. and Hubbard, M.G. (1987). Elective mutism in a missionary family: A case study. *Journal of Psychology and Theology* 15, 291–299.

Beckmann-Murray, R. and Wilson-Huelskoetter, M. (1987). *Psychiatric Mental Health Nursing: Giving Emotional Care* (2nd ed.). Norwalk, CT: Appleton & Lange.

Bednar, R.A. (1974). A behavioral approach to treating an elective mute in the school. *Journal of School Psychology* 12, 326–337.

Bell, P.A., Fisher, J.D., Baum, A. and Greene, T.E. (1990). *Environmental Psychology* (3rd ed.). New York: Holt, Rinehart & Winston.

Bennett, A. (1981). Interruptions and the interpretation of conversation. *Discourse Processes* 4, 171–188.

Berko, D.K. (1960). *The Process of Communication*. San Francisco: Rinehart Press.

Besag, V.E. (1989). *Bullies and Victims: A Guide to Understanding and Management*. Philadelphia: Open University.

Bhide, A.V. and Sprinath, S. (1985). Elective mutism. *British Journal of Psychiatry* 147, 731.

Blanchard, E.B. and Epstein, L.H. (1978). *A Biofeedback Primer*. Reading, MA: Addison-Wesley.

Blos, P. (1962). *On Adolescence: A Psychoanalytic Interpretation*. New York: Macmillan.

Blotcky, M.J. and Looney, J.G. (1980). A psychotherapeutic approach to silent children. *American Journal of Psychotherapy* 34, 487–495.

Bly, R. (1990). *Iron John: A Book about Men*. Reading, MA: Addison-Wesley.

Bozigar, J.A. and Hansen, R.A. (1984). Group treatment of elective mute children. *Social Work* 29(5), 478–480.

Bradley, J.C. and Edinberg, M.A. (1982). *Communication in the Nursing Context*. CT: Appleton-Century-Crofts.

Bradley, S. and Sloman, L. (1975). Elective mutism in immigrant families. *Journal of the American Academy of Child Psychiatry* 14, 510–514.

Brazier, B. and MacDonald, L. (1981). Ethical decision-making in behavioral programming: A continuum of procedures. *Journal of Practical Approaches to Developmental Handicap* 4, 11–13.

Breuer, J. and Freud, S. (1957). *Studies in Hysteria*. New York: Basic Books.

Brickel, C.M. (1981). A review of the roles of pet animals in psychotherapy and with the elderly. *International Journal of Aging and Human Development* 12, 119–128.

Brickel, C.M. (1986). Pet-facilitated therapies: A review of the literature and clinical implementation considerations. *Clinical Gerontologist* 5, 309–332.

Bross, A. (1982). *Family Therapy: A Recursive Model of Strategic Practice*. New York: Methuen.

Brown, B. and Doll, B. (1988). Case illustration of classroom intervention with an elective mute child. *Special Services in the Schools* 5, 107–125.

Browne, E., Wilson, V. and Laybourne, P.C. (1963). Diagnosis and treatment of elective mutism in children. *Journal of the American Academy of Child Psychiatry* 2, 605–617.

Burd, S.F. and Marshall, M.A. (1963). *Some Clinical Approaches to Psychiatric Nursing*. New York: Macmillan.

Burgoon, J.K. and Saine, T. (1978). *The Unspoken Dialogue: An Introduction to Nonverbal Communication*. Boston: Houghton Mifflin.

Burton, A. (1972). *Interpersonal Psychotherapy*. Englewood Cliffs, NJ: Prentice-Hall.

Calhoun, J. and Koenig, K.L. (1973). Classroom modification of elective mutism. *Behavior Therapy* 4, 700–702.

Carr, A. and Afnan, S. (1989). Concurrent individual and family therapy in a case of elective mutism. *Journal of Family Therapy* 11, 29–44.

Cassirer, E. (1946). *Essay on Man*. New Haven: Yale University Press.

Cautela, J.R. (1977). *Behavior Analysis Forms for Clinical Intervention* (Vol. 2). Champaign, IL: Research Press.

Cautela, J.R. and Kastenbaum, R. (1977). A reinforcement survey schedule for use in therapy, training, and research. *Psychological Reports* 20, 115–1130.

Chapman, R.S. and Miller, J.F. (1980). Analyzing language and communication in the child. In R. Schiefelbusch (ed.), *Nonspeech Language*. Baltimore: University Park Press.

Chassan, J.B. (1979). *Research Design in Clinical Psychology and Psychiatry* (2nd ed.). New York: Irvington.

Chethik, M. (1973). Amy: The intensive treatment of an elective mute. *Journal of the American Academy of Child Psychiatry* 12, 482–498.

Ciottone, R.A. and Madonna, J.M. (1984). The treatment of elective mutism: The economics of an integrated approach. *Techniques: Journal of Remedial Education and Counselling* 1, 23–30.

Clark, H.H. and Clark, E.V. (1977). *Psychology and Language: An Introduction to Psycholinguistics*. New York: Harcourt Brace Jovanovich.

Clayton, W.T. (1981). The use of positive reinforcement and stimulus fading in the treatment of an elective mute. *Behavioral Psychotherapy* 9, 25–33.

Cline, T. and Kysel, F. (1988). Children who refuse to speak: Ethic background of children with special educational needs described as elective mute. *Children and Society* 1, 327–334.

Coates, J. (1986). *Women, Men and Language: A Sociolinguistic Account of Sex Differences in Language*. London: Longman.

Colligan, R.W., Colligan, R.C. and Dilliard, M.K. (1977). Contingency management in the classroom treatment of long-term elective mutism: A case report. *Journal of School Psychology* 15, 9–17.

Collins, M. (1977). *Communication in Health*. Saint Louis: C.V. Mosby.

Commission on Professional and Hospital Activities (1978). International classification of diseases, 9th revision, Clinical Modification 9IC9–9–CM. Ann Arbor, MI: Author.

Conrad, R.D., Delk, J.J. and Williams C. (1974). Use of stimulus fading procedures in the treatment of situation specific mutism: A case study. *Journal of Behavior Therapy and Experimental Psychiatry* 5, 99–100.

Cormier, W.H. and Cormier, L.S. (1979). *Interviewing Strategies for Helpers: A Guide to Assessment, Treatment and Evaluation*. Monterey, CA: Brooks/Cole.

Corsini, R.J. (ed.) (1984). *Encyclopedia of Psychology* (Vols. 1–3). New York: John Wiley.

Corson, S.A. and Corson E. (1990). Pets as mediators of therapy in custodial institutions and the aged. In J.H. Masserman (ed.), *Current Psychiatric Therapies* (pp. 277–296). New York: Grune & Stratton.

Coutts, G. (1985). Elective mutism. *Reporter (OECTA)* (November), pp. 36–37.

Crema, J.E. and Kerr, J.M. (1978). Elective mutism: A child care case study. *Child Care Quarterly* 7, 215–226.

Croghan, L.M. and Craven, R. (1982). Elective mutism: Learning from the analysis of a successful case history. *Journal of Pediatric Psychology* 7, 85–93.

Crumley, F.E. (1990). The masquerade of mutism. *Journal of the American Academy of Child and Adolescent Psychiatry* 29, 318–319.

Cunningham, C.E., Cataldo, M.F., Mallion, C. and Keyes, J.B. (1983). A review and controlled single case evaluation of behavioral approaches to the management of elective mutism. *Child and Family Behavior Therapy* 5(4), 25–49.

Dabbs, J.M., Ruback, R.B. and Evans, M.S. (1987). "Grouptalk": Sound and silence in group conversation. In A.W. Siegman and S. Feldstein (eds.), *Nonverbal Behavior and Communication* (2nd ed., pp. 501–520). New York: Lawrence Erlbaum Associates.

Dallmayr, F.R. (1985). *Language and Politics: Why Does Language Matter to Political Philosophy?* London: University of Notre Dame Press.

Daniel, A.E. and Resnick, P.J. (1987). Mutism, malingering, and competency to stand trial. *Bulletin of the American Academy of Psychiatry and the Law* 15(3), 301–308.

Danskin, D.G. and Crow, M.A. (1981). *Biofeedback*. Palo Alto, CA: Mayfield.

Devito, J.A. (1983). *The Interpersonal Communication Book*. New York: Harper & Row.

Dmitriev, V. and Hawkins, J. (1973). Susie Wever used to say a word. *Teaching Exceptional Children* 6, 68–76.

Dowrick, P.W. and Dove, C. (1980). The use of self-modeling to improve swimming performance in spina bifida children. *Journal of Applied Behavior Analysis* 13, 51–56.

Dowrick, P.W. and Hood, M. (1978). Transfer of talking behavior across settings using faked films. In E.L. Glynn and S.S. McNaughton (eds.), *Proceedings of the New Zealand Conference for Research in Applied Behavior Analysis*. Auckland, New Zealand: University of Auckland Press.

Duncan, S. Jr. and Riske, D.W. (1977). *Face-to-face Interaction: Research, Method and Theory*. New York: John Wiley.

Durham, J.D. and Hardin, S.B. (1986). *The Nurse Psychotherapist in Private Practice*. New York: Springer.

Eldar, S., Bleich, A., Apter, A. and Tyano, S. (1985). Elective mutism: An atypical antecedent of schizophrenia. *Journal of Adolescence* 3, 289–292.

Eliade, M. (ed.) (1987). *The Encyclopedia of Religion* (Vol. 15, pp. 5709–591). New York: MacMillan.

Ellsworth, P.C. (1975). Direct gaze as a social stimulus: The example of aggression. In P. Pliner, L. Krames and T. Alloway (eds.), *Advances in the Study of Communication and Affect* (pp. 53–75). New York: Plenum Press.

Elson, A., Pearson, C., Jones, D. and Schumacher, E. (1965). Follow-up study of childhood elective mutism. *Archives of General Psychiatry* 13, 182–187.

Entin, A.D. (1982). Family icons: Photographs in family psychotherapy. In E.E. Abt and I.R. Stuart (eds.), *The Newer Therapies: A Source Book* (pp. 207–227). New York: Van Nostrand Reinhold.

Fassler, J. (1978). *Helping Children Cope*. New York: Free Press.

Fernald, G.M. (1943). *Remedial Techniques in Basic School Subjects*. New York: McGraw-Hill.

Ferster, C.B. and Culbertson, S.A. (1982). *Behavior Principles* (3rd ed.). Englewood Cliffs, NJ: Prentice-Hall.

Fessenden, S.A. (1966). Levels of listening – A theory. In S. Ducker (ed.), *Listening Readings* (pp. 30–32). Metuchen, NJ: Scarecrow Press.

Fishbein, H.D. (1984). *The Psychology of Infancy and Childhood*. Hilldale, NJ: Lawrence Erlbaum.

Forward, S. and Buck, C. (1988). *Betrayal of Innocence: Incest and its Devastation*. New York: Penguin.

Francis, G.M. and Baly, A.J. (1984). Plush animals as therapy in a nursing home. *Clinical Gerontologist* 2, 75–76.

Frey, D.H. (1978). Science and the single case in counseling research. *Personnel and Guidance Journal* 56, 263–268.

Friedman, R. and Karagan, N. (1973). Characteristics and management of elective mutism in children. *Psychology in the Schools* 10, 249–252.

Frieze, I.H., Parsons, J.E., Johnson, P.B., Ruble, D.N. and Zellman, G.L. (1978). *Women and Sex Roles: A Social Psychological Perspective*. New York: W.W. Norton.

Fundudis, B., Kolvin, I. and Garside, R.F. (1979). *Speech Retarded and Deaf Children: Their Psychological Development*. New York: Academic Press.

Furst, A.L. (1989). Elective mutism: Report of a case successfully treated by a family doctor. *Israel Journal of Psychiatry and Related Sciences* 26, 96–102.

Gardner, R.A. (1971). *Therapeutic Communication with Children: The Mutual Storytelling Technique*. New York: Aronson.

Garfinkel, A. (1981). *Forms of Explanation*. New Haven: Yale University Press.

Gartner, A., Kohler, M. and Riessman, E. (1971). *Children Teach Children: Learning by Teaching*. New York: Harper & Row.

Gaylord-Ross, R.J., Weeks, M. and Lipner, C. (1980). An analysis of antecedent, response and consequence events in the treatment of self-injurious behavior. *Education and Treatment of the Mentally Retarded* 15, 35–42.

Giglioli, P.P. (1982). *Language and Social Context: Selected Readings*. New York: Penguin.

Gilliland, B.E., James, R.K., Roberts, G.T. and Bowman, J.T. (1984). *Theories and Strategies in Counselling and Psychotherapy*. Englewood Cliffs, NJ: Prentice-Hall.

Glad, D.D. (1959). *Operational Values in Psychotherapy*. New York: Oxford.

Goldenson, R.M. (ed.) (1984). *Longman Dictionary of Psychology and Psychiatry*. New York: Longman.

Goldman Eisler, F. (1968). *Psycholinguistics: Experiments in Spontaneous Speech*. New York: Academic Press.

Goll, K. (1979). Role structure and subculture in families of elective mutists. *Family Process* 18, 55–68.

Golwyn, D.H. and Weinstock, R.C. (1990). Phenelzine treatment of elective mutism: A case report. *Journal of Clinical Psychiatry* 51, 384–385.

Goodwin, M.H. (1990). *He Said–She Said: Talk as Social Organization among Black Children*. Bloomington: Indiana University Press.

Gorden, R.L. (1969). *Interviewing: Strategy, Techniques and Tactics*. Homewood, Il: Dorsey Press.

Gordon, H. (1983). Asking for feedback from helpers. *Peer Facilitator Quarterly*, 1983, 1, 12.

Green, R.L. (1989). Assessment of malingering and defensiveness by objective personality inventories. In R. Rogers (ed.), *Clinical Assessment of Malingering and Deception* (pp. 123–158). New York: Guilford.

Gregory, R.L. (ed.) (1987). *The Oxford Companion to the Mind*. New York: Oxford University Press.

Grinder, J. and Bandler, R. (1975). *The Structure of Magic: A Book about Language and Therapy*. Palo Alto, CA: Science and Behavior Books.

Haeseler, M.P. (1987). Censorship or intervention: "But you said we could draw what we wanted!" *The American Journal of Art Therapy* 26, 11–20.

Halpern, W.I., Hammond, J. and Cohen, R. (1971). A therapeutic approach to speech phobia: Elective mutism reexamined. *Journal of the American Academy of Child Psychiatry* 10, 94–107.

Harré, R. and Lamb, R. (ed.) (1983). *The Encyclopedic Dictionary of Psychology*. Cambridge, MA: Mit Press.

Harrop, A. (1983). Behavior modification in the classroom. London: Hodder and Stroughton.

Hartmann, D.P. and Hall, R.V. (1976). The changing criterion design. *Journal of Applied Behavior Analysis* 9, 527–532.

Harvey, T., Green, P. and Newton, S. (1985). A rewarding experience. *Nursing Times* 81, 38–39.

Hayden, T.L. (1980). Classification of elective mutism. *Journal of the American Academy of Child Psychiatry* 19, 118–133.

Heimlich, E.P. (1981). Patient as assistant therapist in paraverbal therapy with children. *American Journal of Psychotherapy* 35, 262–267.

Helfer, R.E. (1981, October). *Developmental Deficits Which Limit Interpersonal Skills.* Paper presented at the Newfoundland Conference on Child Abuse, St. John's Newfoundland.

Hesselman, S. (1983). Elective mutism in children 1877–1981. *ACTA Paedopsychiatica* 49(6), 297–310.

Hersen, M. (1982). Single case experimental designs. In A. Bellack, M. Hersen and A. Kazdin (eds.), *International Handbook of Behavior Therapy* (pp. 167–210). New York: Plenum Press.

Hersen, M. and Barlow, D.H. (1976). *Single Case Experimental Designs.* New York: Pergamon.

Hewett, F.M. (1968). *The Emotionally Disturbed Child in the Classroom.* Boston, MA: Allyn & Bacon.

Hill, L. and Scull, J. (1985). Elective mutism associated with selective inactivity. *Journal of Communication Disorders* 18, 161–167.

Hoch, P.H. and Zubin, J. (eds.) (1955). *Psychopathology of Childhood.* New York: Grune & Stratton.

Hoffman, S. and Laub, B. (1986). Paradoxical intervention using a polarization model of cotherapy in the treatment of elective mutism: A case study. *Contemporary Family Therapy* 8, 136–143.

Hollender, M.H. and Ford, C.V. (1990). *Dynamic Psychotherapy: An Introductory Approach.* Washington, DC: American Psychiatric Press.

Homme, L., Csanyi, A.P., Gonzales, M.A. and Rechs, J.R. (1970). *How to Use Contingency Contracting in the Classroom.* Champaign, IL: Research Press.

Horner, T.M. (1985). The psychic life of the young infant: Review and critique of the psychoanalytic concepts of symbiosis and infantile omnipotence. *American Journal of Orthopsychiatry* 55, 324–344.

Jackson, D.D. (1965). Family rules: Marital quid pro quo. In G.D. Erikson and T.P. Hogan (eds.), *Family Therapy: An Introduction to Theory and Technique* (pp. 76–85). Monterey, CA: Brooks/Cole.

Jaffe, J. and Feldstein, S. (1970). *Rhythms of Dialogue.* New York: Academic Press.

Janosik, E.H. and Davies, J.L. (1986). *Psychiatric Mental Health Nursing.* Boston: Jones and Bartlett.

Johnson, W. and Associates (1959). *The Onset of Stuttering.* Minneapolis: University of Minnesota Press.

Jones, R.M. (1970). *System in Child Language.* Cardiff: University of Wales Press.

Kagan, J., Resnick, J.S. and Snidman, N. (1987). The physiology and psychology of behavioral inhibition in children. *Child Development* 58, 1459–1473.

Kagan, J. and Snidman, N. (1991). Infant predictors of inhibited and uninhibited profiles. *Psychological-Science* 2, 40–44.

Kahn, J.S., Kehle, T.J., Jenson, W.R. and Clark, E. (1990). Comparison of cognitive-behavioral, relaxation and self-modeling for depression among middle-school students. *School Psychology Review* 19(2), 196–211.

Kalma, A. (1992). Gazing in triads: A powerful signal in floor apportionment. *British Journal of Social Psychology* 31, 21–29.

Kanfer, F.H. and Gaelick-Buys, L. (1991). Self-management methods. In F.H. Kanfer and A.P. Goldstein (eds.), *Helping People Change: A Textbook of Methods* (4th ed.) (pp. 305–360). New York: Pergamon Press.

Kanfer, F.H. and Saslow, G. (1969). Behavioral diagnosis. In C.M. Franks (ed.), *Behavior Therapy: Appraisal and Status* (pp. 417–444). New York: McGraw-Hill.

Kaplan, S.L. and Escoll, P. (1973). Treatment of two silent adolescent girls. *Journal of the American Academy of Child Psychiatry* 12, 59–72.

Katz, A.M. and Katz, V.T. (1983). *Foundations of Nonverbal Communication*. Carbondale, IL: Southern Illinois University.

Kazdin, A.E. (1982). Methodological strategies in behavior-therapy research. In G.T. Wilson and C.M. Franks (eds.), *Contemporary Behavior Therapy: Conceptual and Empirical Foundations* (pp. 403–442). New York: Guilford Press.

Kehle, T.J. and Gonzales, F. (1991). Self-modeling for children's emotional and social concerns. In P.W. Dowrick (ed.), *Practical Guide to Using Video in the Behavioral Sciences* (pp. 244–255). New York: John Wiley.

Kehle, T.J., Owen, S.V. and Cressey, E.T. (1990). The use of self-modeling as an intervention in school psychology: A case study of an elective mute. *School Psychology Review* 19, 115–121.

Kendon, A. (1967). Some functions of gaze direction in social interaction. *Acta Psychologica* 26, 1–47.

Kerr, M.M. and Strain, P.S. (1979). The use of peer initiation strategies to improve the social skills of children. In A.H. Fink (ed.), *International Perspectives on Future Special Education*. Reston, VA: Council for Exceptional Children.

Key, M.R. (1975). *Paralanguage and Kinesics*. Metuchen, NJ: Scarecrow Press.

Klienbaum, D.G., Kupper, L.L. and Morgenstern, H. (1982). *Epidemiological Research*. Belmont, CA: Lifetime Learning Publications.

Knapp, M.L. (1978). *Nonverbal Communication in Human Interaction* (2nd ed.). New York: Holt-Rinehart & Winston.

Knapp, M.L. (1980). *Essentials of Nonverbal Communication*. New York: Holt-Rinehart & Winston.

Knill, P.J. (1978). *Intermodal Learning in Education and Therapy*. Cambridge, MA: Institute for Arts and Human Development, Lesley College Graduate School.

Kolvin, I. and Fundudis, T. (1981). Electively mute children: Psychological development and background factors. *Journal of Child Psychology and Psychiatry* 22, 219–232.

Krolian, E.B. (1988). "Speech is silvern, but silence is golden": Day hospital treatment of two electively mute children. *Clinical Social Work Journal* 16, 355–377.

Kupietz, S.S. and Schwartz, I.L. (1982). Elective mutism: Evaluation and behavioral treatment of three cases. *New York State Journal of Medicine* 82, 1073–1076.

Labbe, E.E. and Williamson, D.A. (1984). Behavioral treatment of elective mutism: A review of the literature. *Clinical Psychological Review* 4, 273–392.

Lachenmeyer, J.R. and Gibbs, M.S. (1985). The social-psychological functions of reward in the treatment of a case of elective mutism. *Journal of Social and Clinical Psychology* 3, 466–473.

Lachman-Chapin, M. (1983). The artist as clinician: An interactive technique in art therapy. *American Journal of Art Therapy* 23, 13–25.

Landgarten, H. (1975). Art therapy as the primary mode of treatment for an elective mute. *American Journal of Art Therapy* 14, 121–125.

Lazarus, A.A. (1976). *Multimodel Behavior Therapy*. New York: Springer Publishing.

Lazarus, P.J., Gavilo, H.M. and Moore, J.W. (1983). The treatment of elective mutism within the school setting: Two case studies. *School Psychology Review* 12, 467–472.

Leary, M.R., Knight, P.D., Johnson, K.A. (1987). Social anxiety and dyadic conversation: A verbal response analysis. *Journal of Social and Clinical Psychology* 507, 34–50.

Lepper, M.R. and Gilovich, T. (1981). The multiple functions of reward: A social-developmental perspective. In S.S. Brehm, J.M. Kassin and F.X. Gibbons (eds.), *Developmental Social Psychology*. New York: Oxford University Press.

Lesser-Katz, M. (1988). The treatment of elective mutism as stranger reaction. *Psychotherapy* 2, 305–311.

Lewin, B.D. (1968). *The Second Look: The Reconstruction of Personal History in Psychiatry and Psychoanalysis.* Baltimore: John Hopkins.

Lewis, G.K. (1978). *Nurse-Patient Communication* (3rd ed.). Dubuque, Iowa: Wm. C. Brown.

Light, R.J. and Pillemer, D.B. (1984). *Summing Up: The Science of Reviewing Research.* Cambridge, MA: Harvard University.

Lipton, H. (1980). Rapid reinstatement of speech using stimulus fading with a selectively mute child. *Journal of Behavior Therapy and Experimental Psychiatry* 11, 147–149.

Longo, D.C. and Williams, R.A. (1986). *Clinical Practice in Psychosocial Nursing: Assessment and Intervention* (2nd ed.). New York: Appleton-Century-Croft.

Louden, D.M. (1987). Elective mutism: A case study of a disorder of childhood. *Journal of the National Medical Association* 79, 1043–1048.

Lowenstein, L.F. (1979). The result of twenty-one elective mute cases. *Acta Paedopsychiatrica* 45, 17–23.

Lumb, D. and Wolff, D. (1988). Mary doesn't talk. *British Journal of Special Education* 15, 103–107.

Mahl, G.F. (1956). Disturbances and silences in the patient's speech in psychopathology. *Journal of Abnormal and Social Psychology* 53, 1–15.

Mahler, M.S. (1973). On the first three subphases of the separation-individualization process. In Chess, S. and Thomas, A. (eds.), *Annual Progress in Child Psychiatry and Child Development* (pp. 128–138). New York: Brunner/Mazel.

Mahler, M.S. and Glosliner, B.J. (1955). On symbiotic child psychosis. *The Psychoanalytic Study of the Child* 10, 195–212.

Mahler, M.S., Pine, F. and Berman, A. (1975). *The Psychological Birth of the Human Infant.* New York: Basic Books.

Maletzky, B.M. (1974). Behavior recording as treatment: A brief note. *Behavior Therapy* 5, 107–112.

Maltz, D.N. and Borker, R.A. (1982). A cultural approach to male-female miscommunication. In J.J. Gumperz (ed.), *Language and Social Identity* (pp. 196–216). Cambridge: Cambridge University Press.

Marcus, P., Holt, P. and Nagurney, M. (1973). Three teachers/three children. *Instructor* 83, 56–58.

Martin, D.G. (1972). *Learning-Based Client-Centered Therapy.* Belmont, CA: Brooks/Cole.

Martin, G. and Pear, J. (1992). *Behavior Modification: What It Is and How to Do It.* Englewood Cliffs, NJ: Prentice-Hall.

McDonald, E.T. (1980). Early identification and treatment of children at risk for speech development. In R. Schiefelbusch (ed.), *Nonspeech Language.* Baltimore: University Park Press.

McFall, R.M. (1976). Parameters of self-monitoring. In R.B. Stuart (ed.), *Behavioral Self-Management: Strategies, Techniques, and Outcomes.* New York: Brunner/Mazel.

Meagher, P.K., O'Brien, T.C. and Aherne, C.M. (eds.) (1979). *Encyclopedic Dictionary of Religion* (Vols. 1–3). Washington, DC: Corpus Publications.

Meerloo, J.A.M. (1958). *Conversation and Communication.* New York: International Universities Press.

Meijer, A. (1979). Elective mutism in children. *Israel Annals of Psychiatry and Related Disciplines* 17(2), 93–100.

Merleau-Ponty, M. (1945). *Phénoménologie de la Perception.* Paris: Gallimard.

Meyers, S.V. (1984). Elective mutism in children: A family systems approach. *The American Journal of Family Therapy* 12(4), 39–45.

Mook, D.G. (1982). *Psychological Research: Strategy and Tactics.* New York: Harper and Row.

Mora, G., DeVault, S. and Schopler, E. (1962). Dynamics and psychotherapy of identical twins with elective mutism. *Journal of Child Psychology and Psychiatry* 3, 41–52.

Morganstern, K.P. and Tevlin, H.E. (1981). Behavioral interviewing. In M. Hersen and A.S. Bellack (eds.), *Behavioral Assessment: A Practical Handbook* (2nd ed.) (pp. 71–100). New York: Pergamon.

Morin, C., Ladouceur, R. and Cloutier, R. (1982). Reinforcement procedure in the treatment of reluctant speech. *Journal of Behavior Therapy and Experimental Psychiatry* 13, 145–147.

Morris, J.V. (1953). Cases of elective mutism. *Journal of Mental Deficiency* 57, 661–668.

Munford, P.R., Reardon, D., Liberman, R.P. and Allen, P. (1976). Behavioral treatment of hysterical coughing and mutism: A case study. *Journal of Consulting and Clinical Psychology* 44, 1008–1014.

Murray, R.B. and Huelskoetter, M.M.W. (1991). *Psychiatric Mental Health Nursing: Giving Emotional Care*. Norwalk, CT: Appleton & Lange.

Murray, S.O. (1985). Toward a model of members' methods for recognizing interruptions. *Language in Society* 13, 31–41.

Myers, G.E. and Myers, M.T. (1980). *The Dynamics of Human Communication*. New York: McGraw-Hill.

Nash, R.T., Thorpe, H.W. Andrews, M.M. and Davis K. (1979). A management program for elective mutism. *Psychology in the Schools* 16, 246–253.

Nesbit, W. (1991). *Mutilation of the Spirit: The Educational Context of Emotional Abuse*. St. John's: Memorial University of Newfoundland.

Nesbit, W.C. and Hadley, N.H. (1989). *Essential Life Skills for Personal Competence*. Seattle, WA: Special Child Publications.

Nichols, R.G. and Stevens, L.A. (1957). *Are You Listening?* New York: McGraw-Hill.

Nickerson, E.T. and Laughlin, K.O. (ed.) (1982). *Helping Through Action Oriented Therapies*. Amherst, MA: Human Resource Development Press.

Nolan, J.D. and Pence, C. (1970). Operant conditioning principles in the treatment of a selectively mute child. *Journal of Consulting and Clinical Psychology* 35, 265–268.

Norman, A. and Broman, H.J. (1970). Volume feedback and generalization techniques in shaping speech of an electively mute boy: A case study. *Perceptual and Motor Skills* 31, 463–470.

O'Brien, M. (1974). *Communication and Relationships in Nursing*. Saint Louis: C.V. Mosby.

Okum, B.F. (1987). *Effective Helping, Interviewing and Counselling Techniques*. Monterey, CA: Brookes/Cole.

Paniagua, F.A. (1988). A procedural distinction between elective mutism and progressive mutism. *Journal of Behavior Therapy and Experimental Psychiatry* 19, 207–210.

Paniagua, F.A. and Saeed, M.A. (1987). Labeling and functional language in a case of psychological mutism. *Journal of Behavior Therapy and Experimental Psychiatry* 18, 259–267.

Papalia, D.E. and Olds, S.W. (1990). *A Child's World: Infancy Through Adolescence* (5th ed.). New York: McGraw.

Parker, E.B., Olsen, T.F. and Throckmorton, M.C. (1960). Social casework with elementary school children who do not talk in school. *Social Work* 5, 64–70.

Patterson, R.L. (1976). *Maintaining Effective Token Economies*. Springfield, IL: Charles C. Thomas.

Paul, I.H. (1978). *Psychotherapy*. Chicago: University of Chicago Press.

Pennebaker, J. (1990). *Opening Up: The Healing Power of Confiding in Others*. New York: Morrow.

Piersel, W.C. and Kratochwill, T.R. (1981). A teacher-implemented contingency management package to assess and treat selective mutism. *Behavioral Assessment* 3, 371–382.

Pietrofesa, J.J., Hoffman, A. and Splete, H.H. (1984). *Counselling: An Introduction* (2nd ed.). Boston: Houghton Mifflin.

Pigott, H.E. and Gonzales, F.P. (1987). The efficacy of videotape self-modeling in treating electively mute children. *Journal of Clinical Child Psychology* 16, 106–110.

Plummer, S., Baer, D.M. and LeBlanc, J.M. (1977). Functional considerations in the use of procedural timeout and an effective alternative. *Journal of Applied Behavior Analysis* 10, 689–705.

Pope, B., Blass, T., Siegman, A.W. and Raher, J. (1970). Anxiety and depression in speech. *Journal of Consulting and Clinical Psychology* 35, 128–133.

Poyatos, F. (ed.) (1988). *Cross-Cultural Perspectives in Nonverbal Communication.* Lewiston, NY: C.J. Hogrefe.

Pustrom, E. and Speers, R.W. (1964). Elective mutism in children. *Journal of the American Academy of Child Psychiatry* 3, 287–297.

Quinn, K.M. (1988). Children and deception. In R. Rogers (ed.), *Clinical Assessment of Malingering and Deception* (pp. 104–119). New York: Guilford Press.

Rachman, S.J. (1989). *Fear and Courage* (2nd ed.). San Francisco: W.H. Freeman.

Radford, P. (1977). A psychoanalytically-based therapy as the treatment of choice for a six-year-old elective mute. *Journal of Child Psychotherapy* 4, 49–65.

Rasbury, W.C. (1974). Behavioral treatment of elective mutism: A case report. *Journal of Behavior Therapy and Experimental Psychiatry* 5, 103–104.

Ray, W.S. (1964). *The Science of Psychology.* New York: McMillan.

Reed, G.F. (1963). Elective mutism in children: A reappraisal. *Journal of Child Psychology and Psychiatry* 4, 99–107.

Reese, H.W. (1989). Rules and rule-governance: Cognitive and behavioristic views. In S.C. Hayes (ed.), *Rule-governed Behavior: Cognition, Contingencies and Instructional Control* (pp. 3–84). New York: Plenum Press.

Reid, J.B., Hawkins, N., Keutzer, C., McNeal, S.A., Phelps, R.E., Reid, K.M. and Mees, H.L. (1967). A marathon behavior modification of a selectively mute child. *Journal of Child Psychology and Psychiatry* 8, 27–30.

Reid, W.H. (1980). *Basic Intensive Psychotherapy.* New York: Brunner/Mazel.

Resnick, P.J. (1989). Malingering of posttraumatic disorders. In R. Rogers (ed.), *Clinical Assessment of Malingering and Deception* (pp. 84–103). New York: Guilford.

Reynolds, G.S. (1975). *A Primer of Operant Conditioning.* Glenview, IL: Scott Foresman.

Richards, C.S. and Hansen, M.K. (1978). A further demonstration of the efficacy of stimulus fading treatment of elective mutism. *Journal of Behavior Therapy and Experimental Psychiatry* 9, 57–60.

Rifkin, A. (1991). Letter to editor. *Comprehensive Psychiatry* 32, 559–560.

Rimm, D.C. and Masters, J.V. (1974). *Behavior Therapy Techniques and Empirical Findings.* New York: Academic Press.

Roberts, J. (1984). Switching models: Family and team choice points and reactions as we moved from the Haley strategic model to the Milan model. *Journal of Strategic and Systematic Therapies* 4, 40–53.

Robins, L.N. (1966). *Deviant Children Grown Up.* Baltimore: Williams & Wilkins.

Rogers, R. (1989a). Introduction. In R. Rogers (ed.), *Clinical Assessment of Malingering and Deception* (pp. 1–9). New York: Guilford.

Rogers, R. (1989b). Structured interviews and dissimulation. In R. Rogers (ed.), *Clinical Assessment of Malingering and Deception* (pp. 250–268). New York: Guilford.

Rosenbaum, E. and Kellman, M. (1973). Treatment of a selectively mute third-grade child. *Journal of School Psychology* 11, 26–29.

Rosenberg, J.B. and Lindblad, M.B. (1978). Behavior therapy in a family context: Treating elective mutism. *Family Process* 17, 77–82.

Ross, S.B. (1983). The therapeutic use of animals with the handicapped. *International Child Welfare Review* 56, 26–39.

Roszak, T. (1969). *The Making of a Counter Culture.* New York: Doubleday.

Ruzicka, B.B. and Sackin, H.D. (1974). Elective mutism: The impact of the patient's silent detachment upon the therapist. *Journal of the American Academy of Child Psychiatry* 13, 551–561.

Saari, C. (1988). Interpretation: Event or process. *Clinical Social Work Journal* 16, 378–390.

Sachs, J. (1987). Young children's language use in pretend play. In S.U. Phillips, S. Steele and C. Tanz (eds.), *Language, Gender and Sex in Comparative Perspective* (pp. 178–188). Cambridge: Cambridge University Press.

Salfield, D.J. (1950). Observations of elective mutism in children. *Journal of Mental Science* 96, 1024–1032.

Sanok, R.L. and Ascoine, F.R. (1979). Behavioral interventions for childhood elective mutism: An evaluative review. *Child Behavior Therapy* 1, 49–68.

Sathre–Eldon, F.S., Olson, R.W. and Whitney, C.I. (1981). *Let's Talk: An Introduction to Interpersonal Communication*. Glenview, IL: Scott Foresman.

Satir, V. (1972). *Peoplemaking*. Palo Alto, CA: Science and Behavior Books.

Schaefer, C.E. and Reid, S.E. (eds.) (1986). *Game Play: Therapeutic Use of Childhood Games*. New York: John Wiley.

Scherer, K.R. and Ikman, P. (1982). *Handbook of Methods in Nonverbal Behavior Research*. New York: Cambridge University Press.

Schmerling, J.D. and Kerins, M.A. (1987). Stimulating communication in a child with elective mutism: Collaborative interventions. *American Journal of Dance Therapy* 10, 27–40.

Shepard, R. (1971). *Mime: The Technique of Silence*. New York: Drama Book Specialists.

Shreeve, D.F. (1991). Elective mutism: Origins in stranger anxiety and selective attention. *Bulletin of the Menninger Clinic* 55, 491–504.

Sidman, M. (1960). *Tactics of Scientific Research*. New York: Basic Books.

Siegman, A.W. (1978a). The meaning of silent pauses in the initial interview. *Journal of Mental and Nervous Disease* 166, 642–654.

Siegman, A.W. (1978b). The telltale voice: Nonverbal messages of verbal communication. In A.W. Siegman and S. Feldstein (eds.), *Nonverbal Behavior and Communication*. Hillsdale, NJ: Lawrence Earlbaum Associates.

Sigelman, C.K., Budd, E.C., Winer, J.L., Schoenrock, C.J. and Martin, P.W. (1982). Evaluating alternative techniques of questioning mentally retarded persons. *American Journal of Mental Deficiency* 86, 511–518.

Skinner, B.F. (1989). The behavior of the listener. In S.C. Hayes (ed.), *Rule-Governed Behavior: Cognition, Contingencies, and Instructional Control* (pp. 85–96). New York: Plenum Press.

Sloop, E.W. (1975). Parents as behavior modifiers. In W.D. Gentry (ed.), *Applied Behavior Modification*. St. Louis: C.V. Mosby.

Sluckin, A. (1977). Children who do not talk at school. *Child Care, Health and Development* 3, 69–179.

Sluzki, C.E. (1983). The sounds of silence: Two cases of elective mutism in bilingual families. *Family Therapy Collections* 6, 68–77.

Smith, B.O. and Ennis, R.H. (1961). *Language and Concepts in Education*. Chicago: Rand McNally.

Smith, D.R. and Williamson, L.K. (1977). *Interpersonal Communication: Roles, Rules, Strategies, and Games*. Dubuque, Iowa: Wm. C. Brown.

Southworth, P. (1987). Happy talk. *Cambridge Journal of Education* 17, 156–158.

Spotnitz, H. (1986). *Modern Psychoanalysis of the Schizophrenic Patient: Theory of the Technique*. New York: Human Sciences Press.

Stotland, E. (1969). *The Psychology of Hope*. San Francisco: Jossey-Bass.

Straughan, J.H. (1968). The application of parent conditioning to the treatment of elective mutism. In H.N. Sloan and B.D. Macauley (eds.), *Operant Procedures in Remedial Speech and Language Training* (pp. 242–255). New York: Houghton Mifflin.

Straughan, J.H., Potter, W.K. Jr. and Hamilton, S.H. (1965). The behavioral treatment of an elective mute. *Journal of Child Psychology and Psychiatry* 6, 125–130.

Strean, H.S. (1984). The patient who would not tell his name. *The Psychoanalytic Quarterly* 53, 410–424.

Subak, M.E., West, M. and Carlin, M. (1982). Elective mutism: An expression of family psychopathology. *International Journal of Family Psychiatry* 3, 335–344.

Sulzer, B. and Mayer, G.R. (1972). *Behavior Modification Procedures for School Personnel.* Hinsdale, IL: The Dryden Press.

Sundeen, S.J., Stuart, G.W., Rankin, E.D. and Cohen, S.A. (1985). *Nurse-Client Interaction: Implementing the Nursing Process.* St. Louis: C.V. Mosby.

Sutherland, S. (1989). *The International Dictionary of Psychology.* New York: Continuum Publishing Company.

Sutton-Smith, B. and Roberts, J.M. (1971). The cross-cultural and psychological study of games. *International Review of Sport Sociology* 6, 79–87.

Tannen, D. (1990). *You Just Don't Understand: Women and Men in Conversation.* New York: Ballantine.

Tawney, J.W. and Gast, D.L. (1984). *Single Subject Research in Special Education.* Columbus, OH: Charles E. Merrill.

Temple, D. (1988). The contrast theory of why-questions. *Philosophy of Science* 55, 141–151.

Tharp, R.G. and Wetzel, R.G. (1969). *Behavior Modification in the Natural Environment.* New York: Academic Press.

Tinbergen, N. (1974). Ethology and stress diseases. *Science* 185, 20–26.

Touchette, P.E., MacDonald, R.F. and Langer, S.N. (1985). A scatter plot for identifying stimulus control of problem behavior. *Journal of Applied Behavior Analysis* 18, 343–351.

Tough, J. (1985). *Listening to Children Talking.* London: Ward Lock Educational.

Ulmer, R.A. (1976). *On the Development of a Token Economy Mental Hospital Treatment Program.* New York: Hemisphere Publishing.

Van der Kooy, D. and Webster, C.D. (1975). A rapidly effective behavior modification program for an electively mute child. *Journal of Behavior Therapy and Experimental Psychiatry* 6, 149–152.

Van Evra, J.P. (1983). *Psychological Disorders of Children and Adolescents.* Boston, MA: Little, Brown and Company.

Van Fraassen, B. (1980). *The Scientific Image.* Oxford: Claredon Press.

Van Riper, C.G. (1971). *The Nature of Stuttering.* Englewood Cliffs, NJ: Prentice-Hall.

Wack, D.M. (1977). Almost always, never ask why. *Transactional Analysis Journal* 7, 252–253.

Wadeson, H. (1986). The influence of art-making on the transference relationship. *Art Therapy* 3, 81–88.

Wahlroos, S. (1974). *Family Communication: A Guide to Emotional Health.* New York: MacMillan.

Warren, B. (ed.) (1984). *Using the Creative Arts in Therapy.* London: Groom Helm.

Wassing, H.E. (1973). A case of prolonged elective mutism in an adolescent boy: On the nature of the condition and its residential treatment. *ACTA Paedopsychiatica* 40, 75–96.

Weininger, O. (1987). Electively mute children: A therapeutic approach, *The Journal of the Melanie Klein Society* 5, 25–42.

Wergeland, H. (1979). Elective mutism. *ACTA Psychiatrica Scandinavica* 59, 218–228.

Wilkins, R. (1985). A comparison of elective mutism and emotional disorders in children. *British Journal of Psychiatry* 146, 198–203.

Williamson, D.A., Sanders, S.H., Sewell, W.R., Haney, W.R. and White, D. (1977). The behavioral treatment of elective mutism: Two case studies. *Journal of Behavior Therapy and Experimental Psychiatry* 8, 143–149.

Wilson, T.G. and O'Leary, K.D. (1980). *Principles of Behavior Therapy.* Englewood Cliffs, NJ: Prentice-Hall.

Winter, S. (1985a). Julie – A programme with a 14-year-old mute – A case study. *Behavioral Approaches with Children* 9, 8–10.

Winter, S. (1985b). Peer therapy for elective mutism. *Behavioral Approaches with Children* 8, 134–137.

Wolman, B.B. (ed.) (1989). *Dictionary of Behavioral Science* (2nd ed.). New York: Academic Press.

Wong, P.T.P. and Weiner, B. (1981). Why people ask "why" questions and the heuristics of attributional search. *Journal of Personality and Social Psychology* 40, 650–663.

Wright, H.F. (1967). *Recording and Analyzing Child Behavior*. New York: Harper and Row.

Wright, H.L. (1968). A clinical study of children who refuse to speak in school. *Journal of the American Academy of Child Psychiatry* 7, 603–617.

Wright, H.H., Miller, M.D., Cook, M.A. and Littman, J.R. (1985). Early identification and intervention with children who refuse to speak. *Journal of the American Academy of Child Psychiatry* 24, 739–746.

Wulbert, M., Nyman, B.A., Snow, D. and Owen, Y. (1973). The efficacy of stimulus fading and contingency management in the treatment of elective mutism A case study. *Journal of Applied Behavior Analysis* 6, 435–441.

Youngerman, J.K. (1979). The syntax of silence: Electively mute therapy. *International Review of Psychoanalysis* 6(3), 283–295.

Zettle, R.D. and Hayes, S.C. (1982). Rule-governed behavior: A potential theoretical framework for cognitive-behavior therapy. In P.C. Kendall (ed.), *Advances in Cognitive-Behavioral Research and Therapy* (pp. 73–118). New York: Academic Press.

Ziller, R.C. (1981). Self, social, environmental orientation through auto-photography. *Personality and Social Psychology Bulletin* 7, 338–343.

Zondlo, F.C. and Scanlan, J.M. (1983). Elective mutism in a 26-year-old deaf female. *Canadian Journal of Psychiatry* 28, 49–51.

NAME INDEX

SUBJECT INDEX

NEUROPSYCHOLOGY AND COGNITION

The purpose of the Neuropsychology and Cognition series is to bring out volumes that promote understanding in topics relating brain and behavior. It is intended for use by both clinicians and research scientists in the fields of neuropsychology, cognitive psychology, psycholinguistics, speech and hearing, as well as education. Examples of topics to be covered in the series would relate to memory, language acquisition and breakdown, reading, attention, developing and aging brain. By addressing the theoretical, empirical, and applied aspects of brain-behavior relationships, this series will try to present the information in the fields of neuropsychology and cognition in a coherent manner.

Series Editor

R. Malatesha Joshi, *Oklahoma State University, U.S.A.*

Publications

1. P.G. Aaron: *Dyslexia and Hyperlexia.* 1989   ISBN 1-55608-079-4

2. R.M. Joshi (ed.): *Written Language Disorders.* 1991   ISBN 0-7923-0902-2

3. A. Caramazza: *Issues in Reading, Writing and Speaking.* A Neuropsychological Perspective. 1991   ISBN 0-7923-0996-0

4. B.F. Pennington (ed.): *Reading Disablities.* Genetic and Neurological Influences. 1991   ISBN 0-7923-1606-1

5. N.H. Hadley: *Elective Mutism.* A Handbook for Educators, Counsellors and Health Care Professionals. 1994   ISBN 0-7923-2418-8

6. W.C. Watt (ed.): *Writing Systems and Cognition.* Perspectives from Psychology, Physiology, Linguistics, and Semiotics. 1994   ISBN 0-7923-2592-3

KLUWER ACADEMIC PUBLISHERS – DORDRECHT / BOSTON / LONDON